No Handicaps

The Life Philosophy of Champion Armless Golfer Tommy McAuliffe,

Edited By Tom McAuliffe II

NEXT STOP PARADISE
PUBLISHING
Ft. Walton Beach, Florida, USA

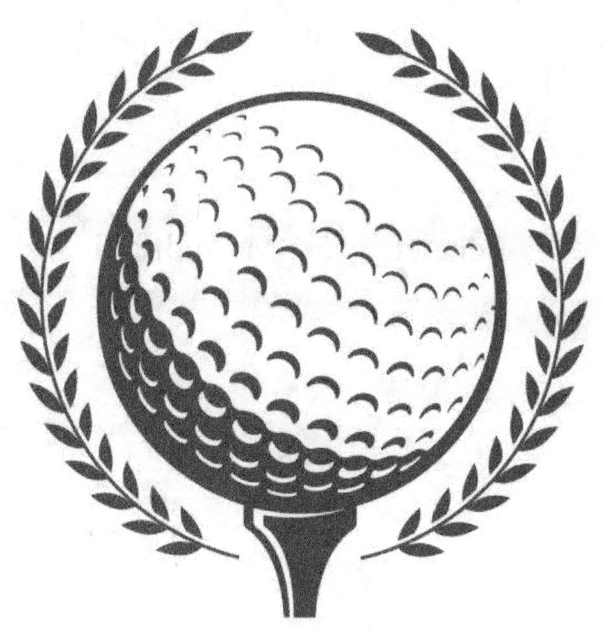

No Handicaps

The Life Philosophy of Champion Armless Golfer Tommy McAuliffe

Printed in the United States of America.
Third Edition - Fall 2024
First Written in 1938

For more information email:
BookInfo@nextstopparadise.com

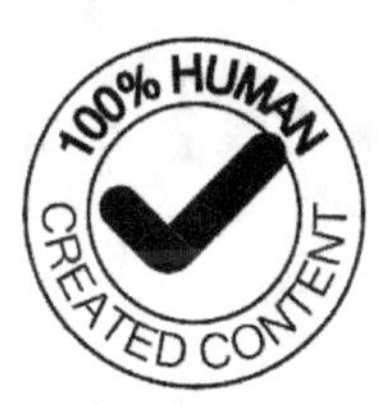

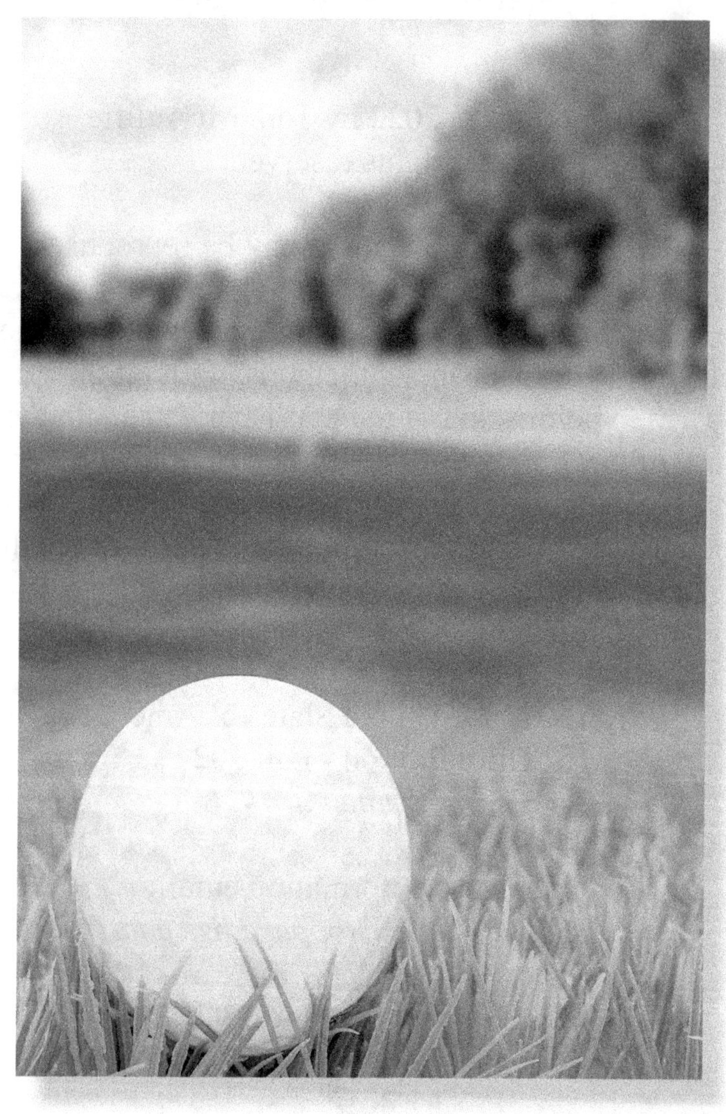

TABLE OF CONTENTS

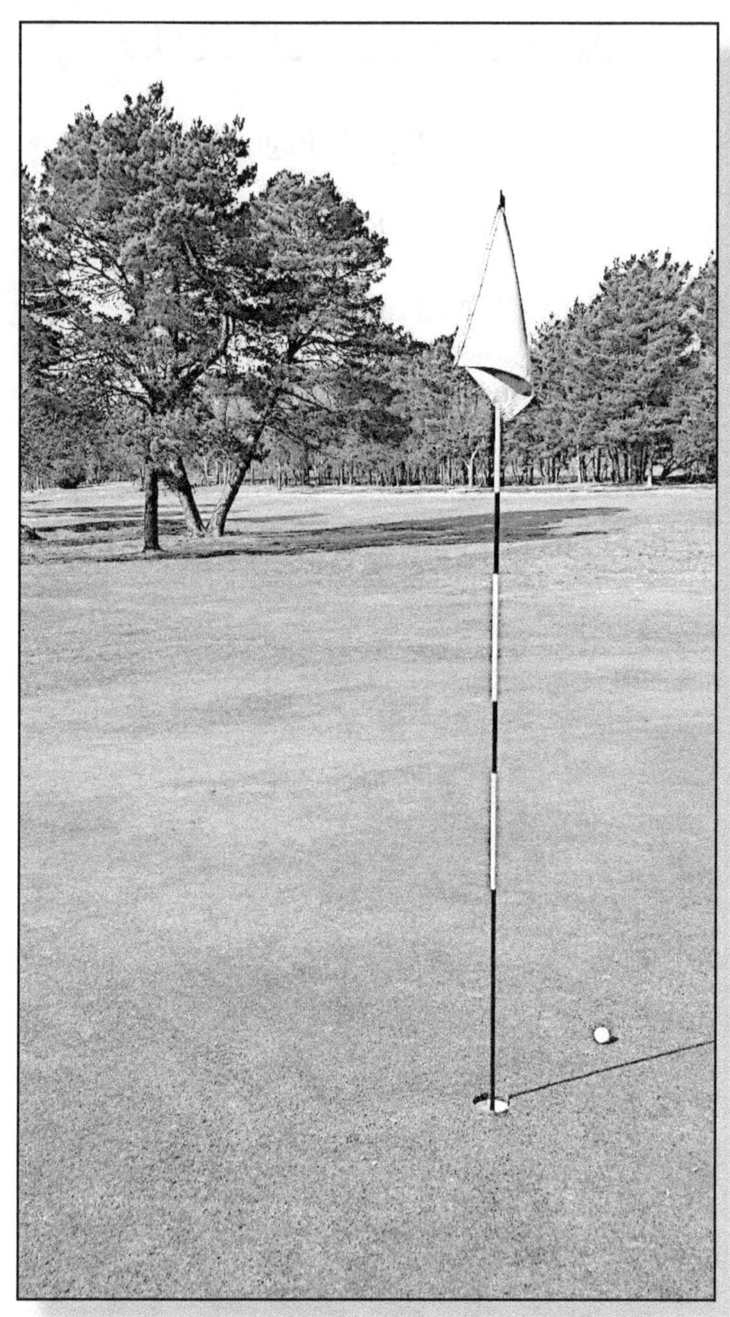

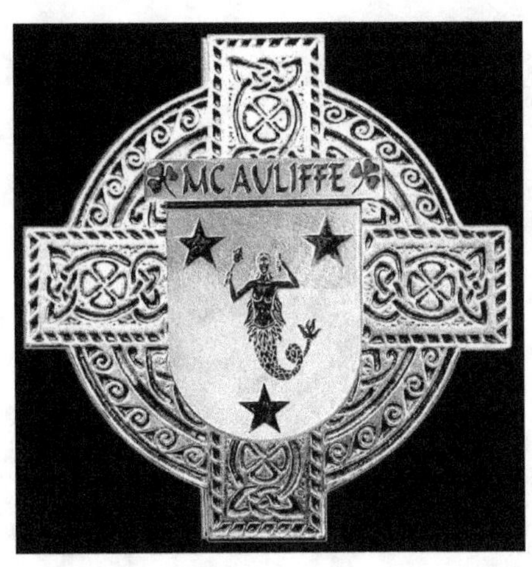

<u>Dedication</u>

To those that believe they have
a handicap… may they come to
see that any limitation can be
overcome with effort
and positive thinking.

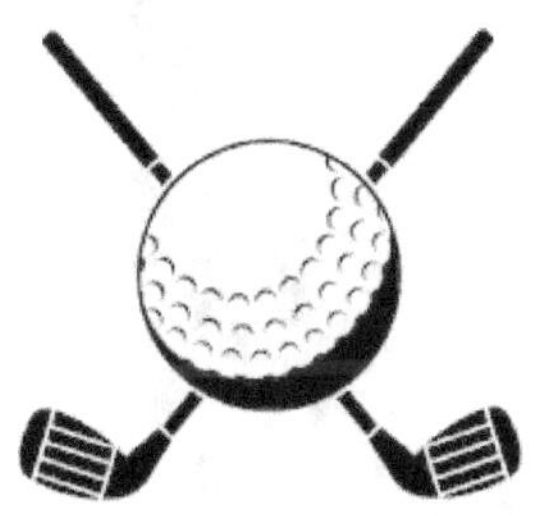

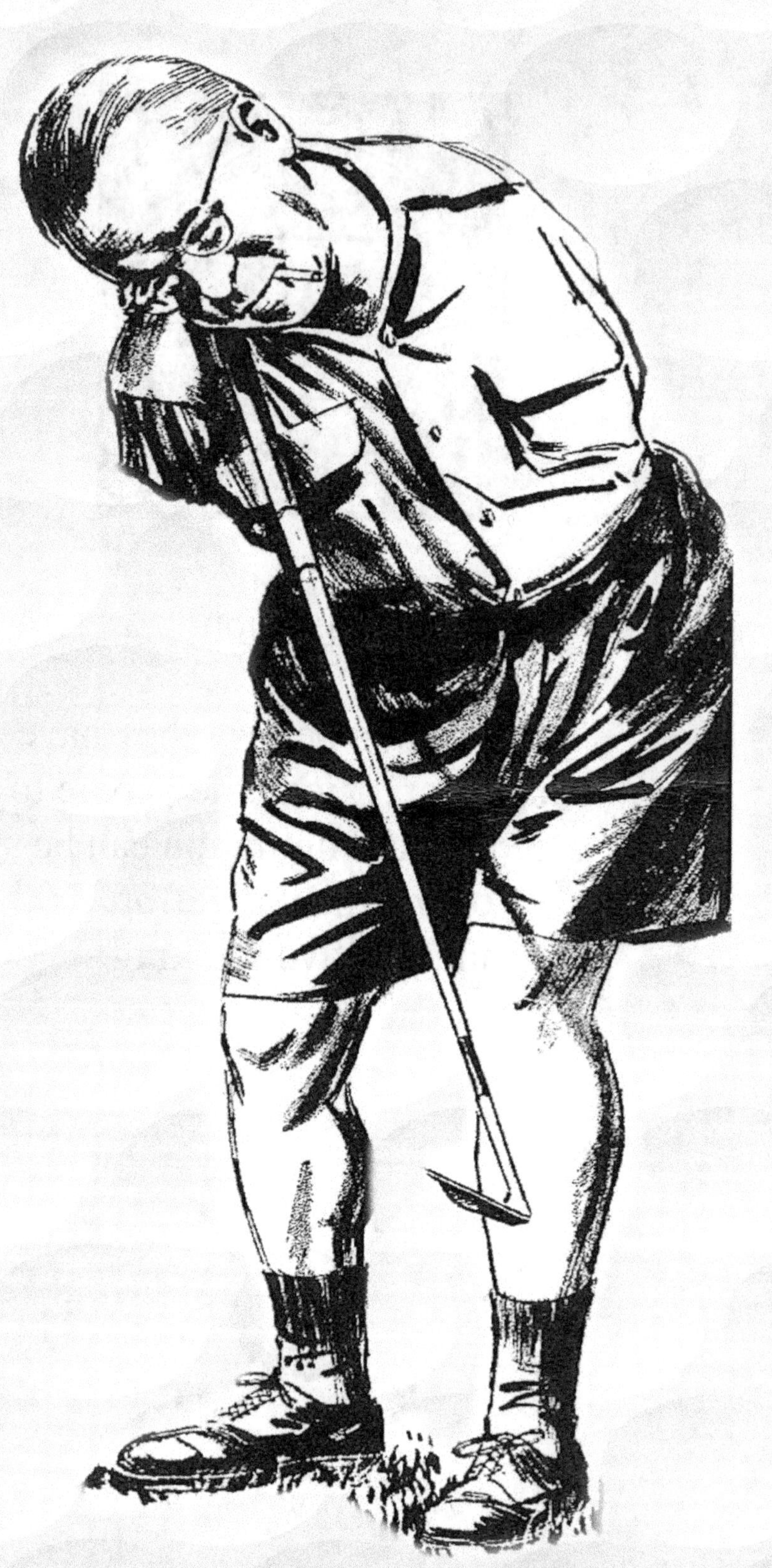

PREFACE

No Handicaps -*The Life Philosophy of Champion Armless Golfer Tommy McAuliffe*, is the uplifting true-life philosophy from a book first written in 1937 by him and edited by yours truly his grandson, Tom Patrick McAuliffe II. One of the original positive-thinking proponents his "No Handicaps" approach has touched thousands of people via articles, appearances and broadcasts back in the day. It was at this time that Dr. James Allen's book "As a Man Thinkth' a forerunner of the Positive thinking movement was published and it was a must read in the McAuliffe household.

Among his accomplishments:

•Played with Golf Legends Walter Hagan, Arnold Palmer and Olympian Bobby Jones.

•Once chipped 282 golf balls into a bushel basket from 25 feet away without missing.

•Played Golf in 49 states, Australia, Canada in one year.

•Promoted laws and testified before Congress on rehabilitation and the physically disabled.

•Designed trick golf shots that have yet to be duplicated.

Author, on-air Radio Host, Public Speaker, Newspaper Reporter, Writer and Magazine Publisher, Farmer, Father, Golfer. Tommy McAuliffe's life outlook of overcoming tragedy with grit and humor via Golf and the will power of the mind proves his theory that 'the only real handicap in life is a mental one!' Talk about self-help! It can benefit all who read it. A leader in the fight for equal rights for the disabled, his inspiring outlook and 'tough love' will delight Golfer and non-Golfer alike!

Think of this as a sort of mental training manual for not just Golf but for life. These are his words, not mine, and written from the heart so long ago yet his lesson are still timely today. These are Tommy McAuliffe's 'Life Lessons' may they help you in life and on the Golf Course. Here's hoping you will use these lessons and soon be on the Fairways of life towards your own hole in one!

Tom

Fall 2024

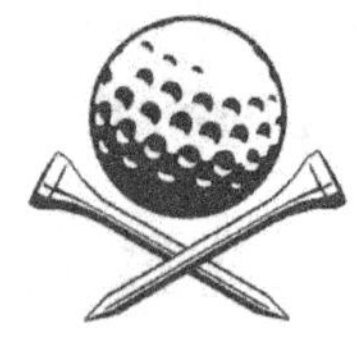

PROLOGUE

"If you worry about the ones you miss, you gonna keep missing them. Remember Tommy the most important shot in golf is always the next one!"
Walter Hagen, Traverse City, MI. 1949

I was born in Buffalo, New York on July 13, 1893, the oldest of five children, and my arms were amputated just below the shoulder after being run over by a street car in 1902 at the age of nine. I have indeed been fortunate and blessed in life and in golf. I have played with the greats including Bobby Jones and Walter Hagan and many other noted golfers who have won national and international golf tournaments. Being able to play is a gift and I remember my first round like it was yesterday…

My first 18 holes resulted in 138 strokes and that was back in 1908 as a Caddy. My lowest score at that time was 108 strokes. I stopped swinging clubs professionally in 1914 and did not really hold another club as a pro until 1928 when I went into Vaudeville. I traveled the world and have enjoyed entertaining audiences around the country from the Paramount Theater in New York City to the Orpheum theater in LA. During the 1932, full-time Vaudeville tour, I played 262 rounds of golf on 260 different courses with an average stroke per round of 90. My lowest score in golf is 82, (a score he made three times; in 1929 at the Royal Queensland course

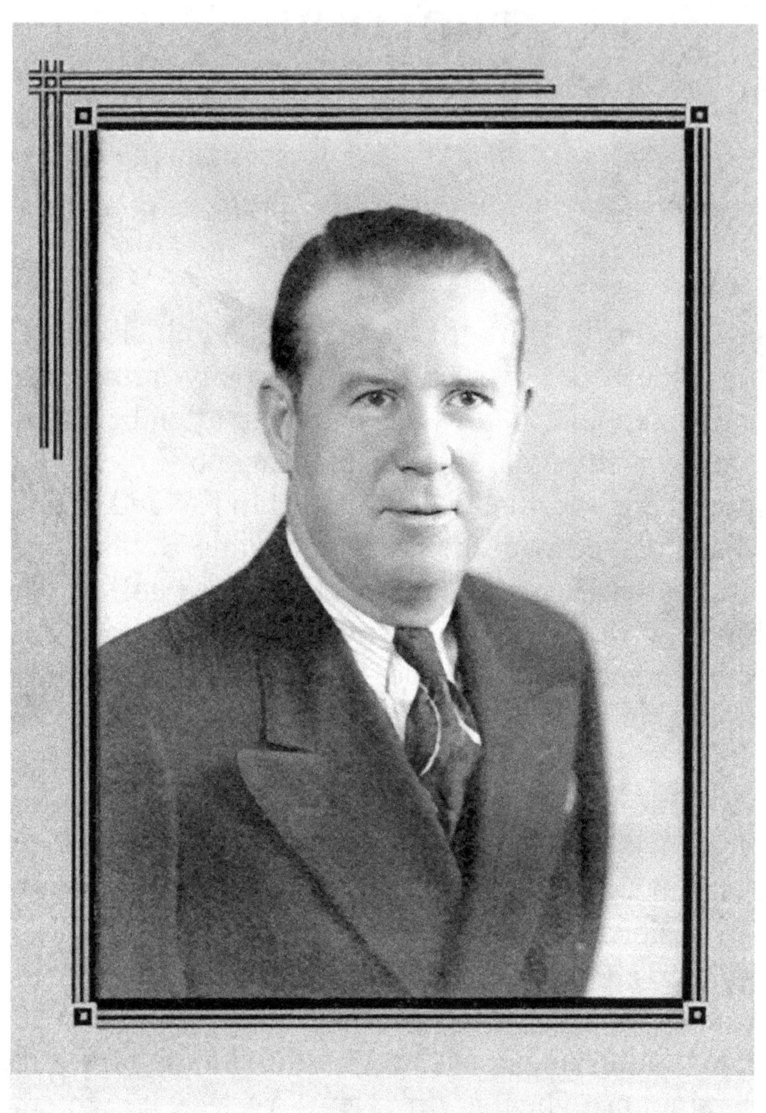

in Brisbane Australia, in 1931 with the Erie Downs Golf Club in Canada and again in 1935 at the Lancaster Country Club in New York). I came close again in 1953 at Plum Hollow Golf Club just outside Detroit. Both are challenging PAR 5 golf courses.

Going to Capitol Hill to testify before Congress and assist in getting action on bills about Rehabilitation was always an honor. The game of Golf has not only been fun and profitable through the years it has taught me valuable life lessons. It's been essential in establishing the mental discipline to overcoming losing both arms and the development of the "No Handicaps" philosophy.

In Golf parlance to "call a Mulligan" is to ask for a do-over. In looking back at my life I hope you can see that instead of quitting life when the streetcar took my arms I simply called a 'Mulligan' and just decided to do my life over. Realizing as I do that success goes to the fighter and with the sound of screeching metal wheels from the train still fresh in my mind even now years later, I vow every day with a determined grin, to simply start all over again. You can too… because I believe there's no handicap in life, except a mental one!

Tommy

Tommy McAuliffe
The Commonwealth Club
Richmond, VA
1957

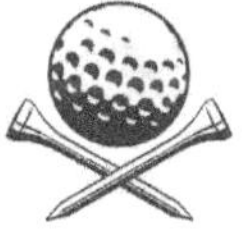

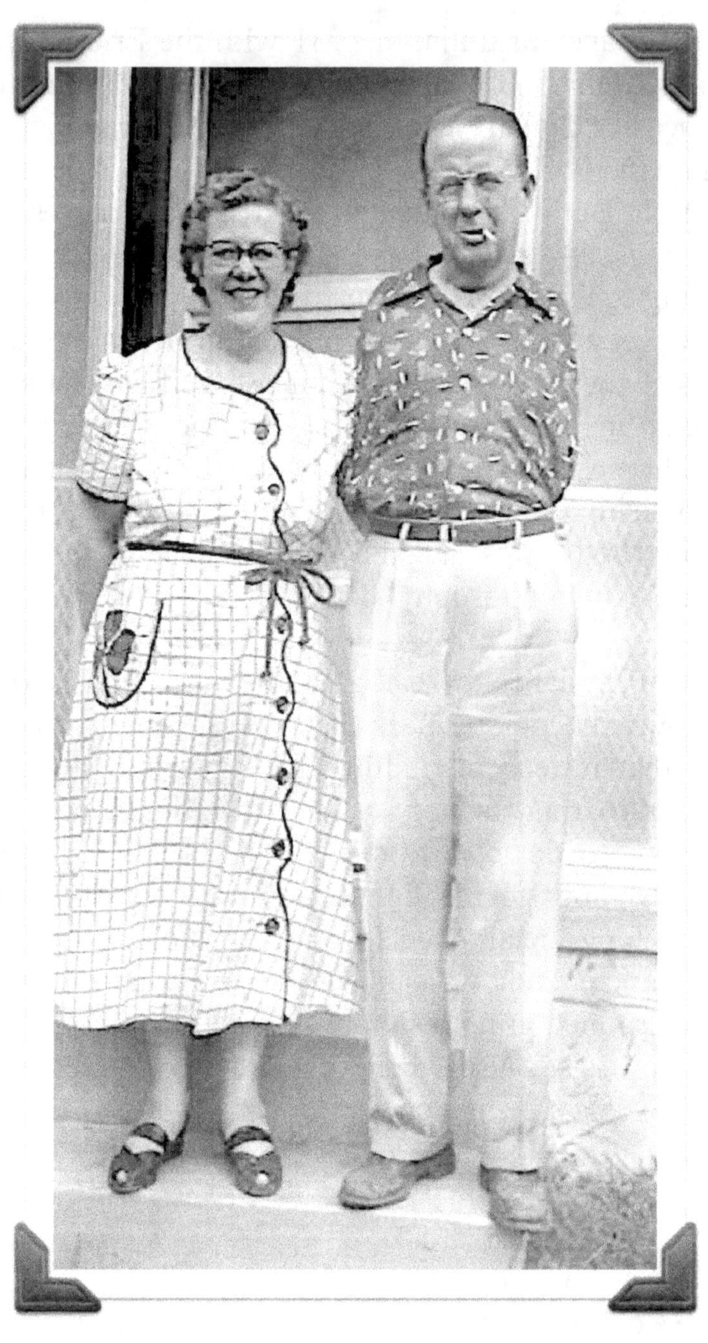

Mr. & Mrs. McAuliffe, Circa 1958

CHAPTER 1

The Two M's
The Importance of Family

*"To find a man's true character,
play golf with him."*
P.G. Wodehouse

*"Golf and sex are the only things you can
enjoy without being good at."*
Jimmy Demerit

People who endeavor to serve others in this struggling world and those who accomplish worthwhile things and amount to something in life have always had some inspiring support behind them. In proving my no handicaps philosophy I claim no exception because my dose of inspiration has been two fold... Without my Mother and my wife Marguerite, my efforts on the golf course, in the media and in helping others including writing this humble volume would not have been possible.

Mother! To be a Mom is one of God's choicest blessings in life. It blessed me with a wonderful Mother in every sense of the word. 'If God wanted you, he would have called you when you were hurt.' This was always my Mom's reminder to me whenever we talked. During those periods in one's life when the feeling of bitter rebellion, resentment and dissatisfaction make their untimely appearance, my Mom's support and guidance was like a tonic but she also made it clear that no sympathy would be forthcoming. Mom always used to say; "He doesn't give you a cross without the strength to carry it." Because of her having an undying faith that God left me here for a specific purpose, I fought on and learned to never take no for an answer. If a thing I wanted or was trying to accomplish was right, I simply chose to believe that God would give me the strength to accomplish it.

Mom's encouragement and empathy never bordered on sympathy, and she wisely allowed me to experience things on my own firsthand. Taking care of Robert, my son, his Mother and his three sisters was indeed a big assignment; like teeing off on a windy day. Life is certainly a colossal task sometimes, a trying problem at best. But what worthwhile subject or endeavor in life is not just that?

I enjoy the struggle although it is disheartening, but it's all part of life and the trick is to find the 'sweet spot'. That's the special part of the club or ball that when you hit it just right sends an almost spiritual ringing to your bones. In writing 'No Handicaps', my purpose is to show that nothing is impossible. A proper mental attitude and follow through, and the principles learned in this crazy game can help both the physically perfect and the imperfect to achieve the most out of life regardless of station or condition. My goal is to spread the gospel that 'there is no handicap in life except a mental one!' But let me get back to Mothers, yours and mine. We have undoubtedly caused her many heartbreaks and many a sleepless night undeservingly so. We would do well to repair any damage and let our mothers know how special they are and how important their support can be. Do it before it's too late. You might also hit your knees and pray that the man upstairs forgives you for the many undeserving heartaches you have caused her. My Mom meant a lot to me.

Although I am the oldest in the family, she always let me know I was her 'baby boy'. The second most important relationship a man has with a woman in life other than his Mother is with his wife. Marguerite, my darling wife, has been my second full dose of inspiration and reality. In her I have found God's angel on earth and a wonderful helpmate. I can truly say that she has no equal and that I am the luckiest man on planet earth. From the day we were married many years ago, as I write this, she has not allowed me to become discouraged for one second. She has made my problems her problems and has counseled me wisely and not quickly. A cheery presence and she backs me up in every wish, desire and attempt to gain the heights of happiness and success.

Our home exudes her wholesomeness, and her motherly instinct creates a true win-win atmosphere. She is more than any man could wish for. She has helped me become a better man, a better businessman, a better communicator and, believe it or not, a better Golfer. Men really owe everything to their wives.

Many times when you return home from the office or shop, you may greet your wife with a frown or a sulk. What if you had a tough day at work where everything went wrong-what about her day? It's not fair play to blame it all on your wife or take it out on her… but how many times do we? Remember, she may have had a trying day in her workshop doing for you and for your children. She deserves consideration. Don't cuss and stew because the toast may be a little too brown or because your dinner is not on the table before you even wash. Keep in mind it's not the easiest job in the world to be a wife and a mother. Before entering the house, stand by the door and count to 10 and then put a big smile on your manly face and enter with a big 'hello darling' and give her a big kiss and a hug.

Don't be afraid to show affection. This has been a challenge for me and you're not a sissy by doing so. A smile and a laugh, regardless of how tough and trying the day was, are always a good tonic to give. History proves that, in the early days, they forced the Japanese to smile. If they failed to smile, they were punished. Sometimes I think it's a pity such a law does not exist today throughout the world. An old Japanese saying is worthy of your thoughts; "He who laughs and smiles away, the little trials of life today, will live to laugh and smile away, the greater trials of another day. " In my travels around the world, people have praised me for what I was with a golf club, but the real credit belongs to my Mom and my wife because their faith, hope, tenacity and womanly resourcefulness completely encompasses and definitely surpass's mine. May you be fortunate enough to have the support of a similar caddy in your corner, as it makes a world of difference.

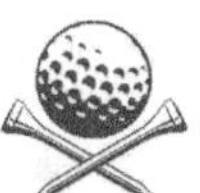

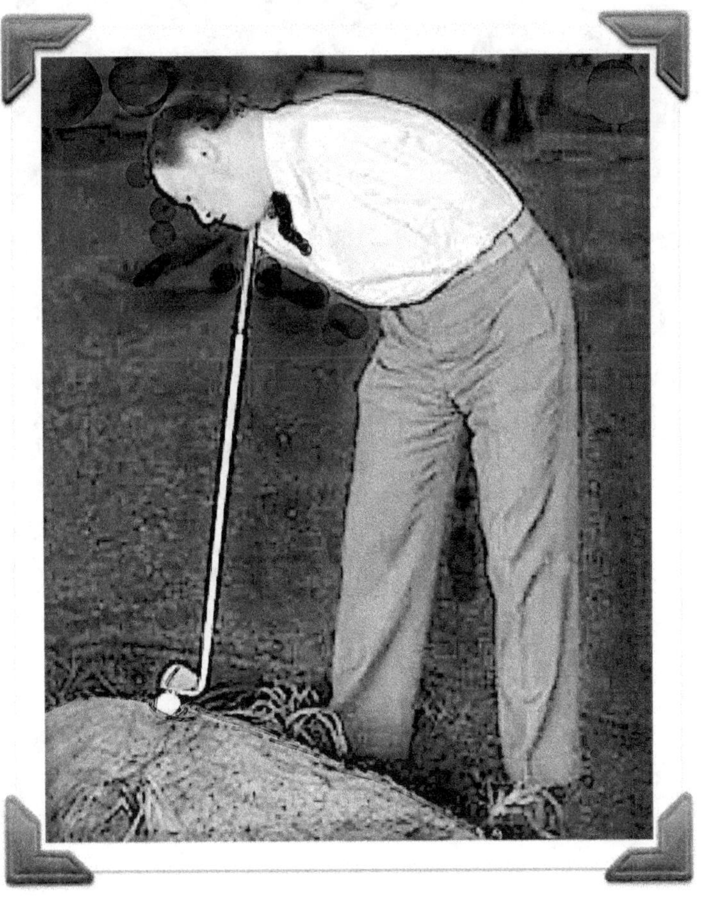

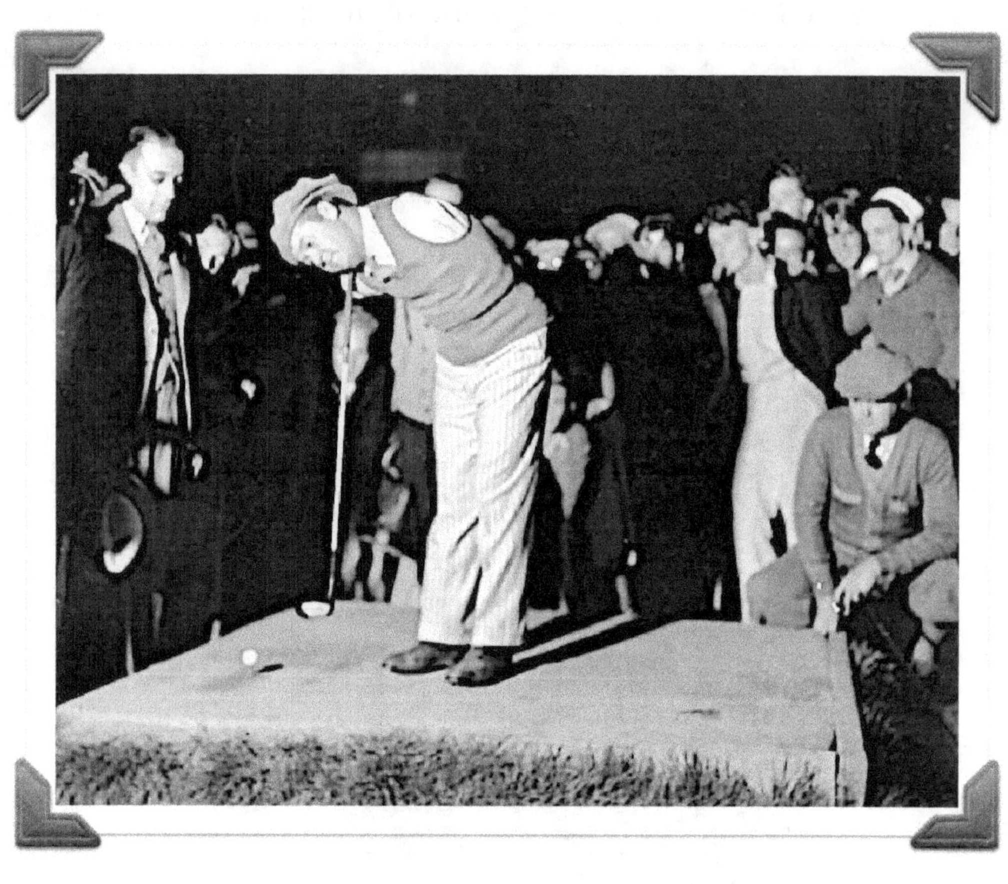

CHAPTER 2

The Mental Attitude
Mind Over Matter

*"They call it golf because all the other
four-letter words were taken!"*
Ray Floyd

A Physical handicap does not mean, should not mean, oblivion in business, society or athletics, nor in life… not anymore. It wasn't always that way. Yet today there are still thousands who think and really believe that a man or a woman with a physical defect is helpless. Nothing could be further from the factual truth. And on the flip-side of that coin are some mental shortcoming or blockage hinders people who are fully able-bodied yet. For many years, it has been my pleasure indeed my privilege to express my thoughts upon the subject of handicapped people before civic and community clubs, chambers of commerce, industrial schools and colleges and visiting and speaking directly with crippled children's institutions. My mission was and is simple with a definite purpose… To spread the unadulterated truth that there is no handicap in life except a mental one and how the lessons I learned in Golf helped me overcome losing both arms and made me a better human being.

In speaking before organizations and over the airwaves and in my writings, the reader will find that I have no personal ax to grind. My pleadings are for and in the interest of the other fellow. People who through a lack of education, circumstances and environment have not secured the truly good life outlook because of the lack of a proper mental attitude. I endeavor to show each that they have no handicap. Your clubs are the same as mine, your ball just as round. My Philosophy on this is self realized. I don't need to have a PhD to know that these principles work. I have lived with the problems of being physically challenged since the accident at nine. Through the firm belief that the mind can overcome almost any handicap, I have been able to do the impossible and at least in some small way, to gain a passing mark in life. What I have experienced and what I have tried to do in proving no handicaps is exactly what every physically affected man and woman must do and learn in order to accomplish things for themselves. The same medicine, in equal dose, pertains to those who are mentally rather than physically challenged.

Let's get the full picture; I am an armless man of modest means and I'm considered by most of modern society to be helpless. Losing both arms was, suffice to say, a life altering experience. One minute I had two arms and the next minute I didn't. Sometimes some people think that it's rather trite when I say these things and you may rightfully ask what steps I took to overcome this tragedy. The very first thing I did was to develop a philosophy of life which can best be summarized in two sentences: First, make the best use of the physical factors I had left (use your best swing). And second, to give my mind the best discipline and training I could get and afford (play often). Following this philosophy, I immediately set about learning to do without the use of arms the things other people could do with a set of arms. It may sound corny to some, but deciding to do a thing really is half the battle. To achieve the second principal in my new philosophy, it became my personal slogan to 'never take no for an answer'.

Going a step further, I find there are three problems a "handicapped" person must face in overcoming their limitations;

1) The first thing is that you must build up and maintain within yourself a large reserve of courage, determination, and belief in self.

2) The problem of securing adequate education and training for a job able to support yourself must be job one.

3) The ability to convince a prospective employer that you can do an honest day's work for an honest day's pay despite any physical limitation.

Fair and equal employment will become the law of the land and none too soon!

So how can a handicapped person build up a reserve of courage and determination? It may sound overly simplified, but success, like happiness, is really just a state of mind. Isn't it? Almost any handicapped person can look about himself and see many others who are more seriously handicapped than they are. Yet they have, despite their handicaps, become useful and happy people. This is equally true of the physically perfect and the opposite is also equally true of people who were born with exceptional gifts of intellect and money yet are unhappy.

Fortunately, hope springs eternal in the human heart and mind. It may sound a little shopworn but I have found that most people are as happy as they make up their minds to be. When a Golfer stops trying for a hole in one every time, their score improves, as does their enjoyment of the game. And this is a simple point that is often overlooked. If the handicapped person is willing to work and hope, the little successes he or she attains will give way to more confidence and with this newfound confidence will come courage and determination to achieve even greater successes.

The trouble with physically challenged people who fail is that they give up too easily. Same is true of those who are new to the game of Golf. They lack perseverance. And this is just as true of the physically complete individual who quits when just one more effort could've led to success. Of course, every person having a physical imperfection, as well as those with no disability, needs these fine and necessary attributes.

Here is where the work of vocational rehabilitation steps in to fill the gap, whereas the physically fit they must do things for themselves. What is vocational rehabilitation you ask? No, it's not some new political party or a new breakfast food, it is a complex mindset which comprises several steps in helping to fit the disabled person for and place them in gainful employment. It's no secret that in American business, we do not give the disabled an equal opportunity on the job front. A few handicapped individuals of general intelligence always seem to get good financial backing unaided, but many must find a way that leads to success with no real help. However, the average physically handicapped person without guidance does not know how to make the adjustments to his combined mental and remaining physical abilities to the requirements of commerce and industry.

All the factors may be present in his or her life situation to develop a feeling of discouragement which aggravates the physical handicap itself and certainly to weaken the desire to make any great effort on his or her own behalf. The result is inevitable in that a spiral occurs, a condition of a dependence upon others, first upon immediate family and then upon society at large. Sadly, after a while, it becomes an ingrained mindset.

True rehabilitation means a job and a chance to live as nearly a normal life as the physical imperfection will allow. Handicapped people do not court nor do they need sympathy from others; empathy perhaps, but sympathy? Never. Knowing this, you readily inquire; what help from others do handicapped people need and require? Most of us, in order to become fully useful and healthy citizens, only need an opportunity. Their mental attitude clearly shows they need encouragement, guidance, and counsel. They need an enlightened interest by the public that will not only expect handicapped people to work but will make it possible for them to get education and training to prepare them for work. In like manner, they need genuine interest by employers to employ handicapped people on their merits as productive workers rather than on any basis of charity. With such an assumption and deep-rooted belief, you may honestly ask, "do handicapped people make capable efficient and dependable workers?" Yes! is the undisputed answer. And like it or not, as the war ends, we will have thousands upon thousands of men and women who have served our country and have come home missing arms and legs.

From my experience and study there are two points in strong favor of giving the handicapped a job and that every fair-minded employer should consider: first, when a person loses one or more bodily members or functions the natural law of compensation and necessity develop pronounce skills in using those functions remaining. Second, because a handicap limits one field of activity, a handicapped worker is more likely to stick to the first job, which promises success and hence is more likely to be a loyal and permanent employee.

On the Golf course, the correlation is being ready to play by having the fundamentals down so that when

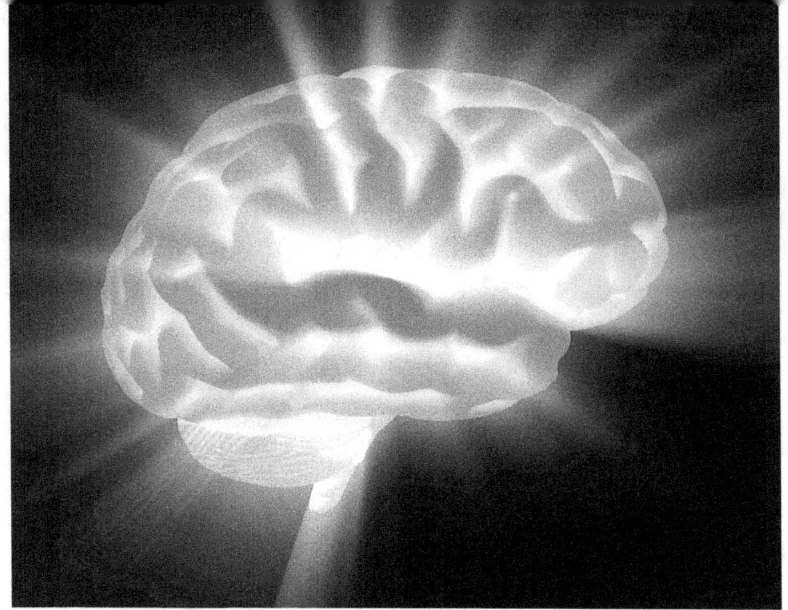

the opportunity comes, you will be ready. And equality of opportunity demands that the physically handicapped be ready, and of course leaders in industry and business should realize the economic value of using handicap workers within their organizations. It's simply good business.

I have a deep personal interest in the other fellow. My chief aim is to spread this gospel and wisdom to the physically handicapped who may be overcome by a negative mindset. A handicap does not have to prevent a person from fully taking part in life. A handicap does not prevent a person from participating in the social, economic, and political activities of his community. My experiences show clearly that people with physical scars at the very outset must learn to do things for self. The proper mental attitude towards life makes the difference.

What is the mental attitude one should have towards life? And what is it my advice? My ideas and experiences have become deep-seated beliefs about the life it has forced me to live. It is not a plan but may be called a humble philosophy of allowing no handicaps. Almost anyone can do what he or she determines to do, but of course, the greater the disability, the harder it is to stand and compete with persons of superior physical abilities. But I say sheer grit and determination can accomplish that more sheer mind power than most people realize.

Sometimes truisms are so simple we look right past them. A disabled person should fully develop the resources left them and entirely ignore those they lack. This is hard medicine to take but believe me it can be done. I know because I have done it. My advice to those who have been informed is to make the best use of the abilities they possess and learn to do things for themselves as soon as possible after the accident.

There may come a day when machines can be attached to replace these arms and legs, but that day is far off. (*Keep in mind this is written in 1937-38 long before modern prosthetics-Ed*) I have found that we would do well to cultivate a spirit of 'I can' and 'I will' and learn to smile… because it's an asset no man can afford to be without. Ever notice you simply feel better when you smile? I have found these life lessons and rehabilitation principles directly through the instructive game of Golf; Concentration, Repetition and perhaps most importantly… Faith.

CHAPTER 3

The Tee Off
Getting Started is Half the Fight

"There are no shortcuts on the quest for perfection."
Ben Hogan

I have a big sign on my bathroom mirror that I see first thing in the morning every day. It says 'there is no handicap in life except a mental one!' I have come to believe this to be true in every respect and over every condition, so it will be my humble aim to prove to you this life outlook called 'No Handicaps'. I found these principles helpful with both my rehabilitation and my life as well as in the sport of Golf. It is a mental sport… and I have found that playing Golf requires not just physical strength and prowess but a strong mental game as well.

As I write this, it was almost 60 years ago that I first met… me! Thomas P McAuliffe, but the Tommy of that distant day is not the same man whom you and I know today. Many things have occurred during these intervening years which have definitely, yes completely, shaped and changed my life and my knowledge of self. And the constant thread through it all is and was Golf and… God.

Friday, July 13 is my birthday. It was on this day that I became the first son of Irish parents. Buffalo, New York, the 13th largest city in America, was the scene of my early life. Two poor struggling parents formed part of my heritage. My father was a City Fireman, one of the few jobs available for Irish immigrants.

Being a chip off the old block, I too have become a different sort of fighter. For nine years, my life was normal, carefree, and like any young boy, I did everything the other kids of my age did. We got into some trouble when we raided my mom's kitchen or made raids to forbidden fruit orchards. Ready for everything and anything, I was a kid in every sense of the word and Mom or a neighbor would've warmed my bottom proper if they could've laid hands upon me!

But I was pretty much a normal kid with dreams of being a professional Baseball Player or Golfer. My early childhood is still vivid. I recall the way we used to sneak into the old swimming hole, only to be chased out by the farmer. Turning the sprinklers on at the local golf course in the middle of the night so that we could cool off, then being chased and sometimes even getting caught, was half the fun. I remember once having to go home without clothing… boy, was my face red and soon my hind-end was as well.

Then, like a thief in the black of night, an incident occurred which changed my life forever. They say that success in life is measured in whole or in part by the deeds one has accomplished. To me, it is further supplemented when its pathway is seemingly insurmountable with barriers. In the blink of an eye, a boy of nine was deprived of both arms just below the shoulder. It seems that I had reached the first high barrier in my brief life.

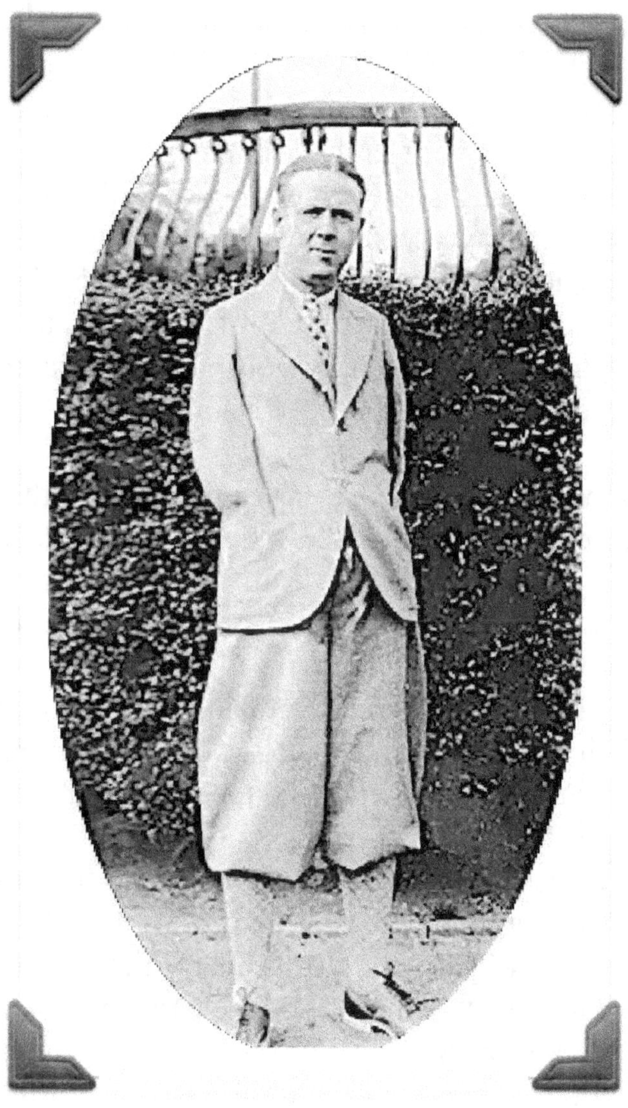

Dapper Duds in 1927

Suddenly, I was different from nine years earlier. There I was armless, but what could I do about it? That my arms would never grow again was certain. I had sense enough to realize that, and the doctors did too. At first I cried to appease my childish heart as I fully realize that I could no longer play and do the things of days gone by.

Family, relatives and friends considered me unfortunate, and some even suggested that it was a shame I had survived. However, over the years, I realize such thoughts depend entirely on one's point of view, one's mental attitude, if you will, and after the crying ended, I simply got mad. How dare they think I can't compete because I don't have two arms!

Born that day, deep in my heart, was a spirit that was to become unconquerable. Initially, my battle was a veritable fight against death itself. Despite the Streetcar's amputation of both arms close to the shoulder socket, I had survived. There were many other physical challenges, but in the end I cheated the Grim Reaper. Little did I know that the mental battle that lay ahead would be ten times as hard.

With arms gone never to return, truly, it was the most discouraging future a person would ever have to face. I had to console myself to this new reality with courage, which is a true characteristic of the Irish race. Energy and ambition were still embedded in my boy's heart and soul. I was determined to make a fight of it to the best of my ability with what I had left. If I was to go down, I was going down swinging! I was determined to fight to have a good life with all the abilities that God had left me. That I would never and again indulge in 'normal' activities and play in the same way failed to put a damper on my spirit. I must and would carry-on, I said to myself… over and over and over. Naturally, at the beginning, disgruntled, disheartened and dissatisfied with my lot, the impatience of youth had me paint a picture that this was always the way it was always going to be (I could not see the Flag on the green!).

At first I was supersensitive and would cry upon the slightest provocation, silly when I think of it today. Regardless of circumstances, I could not be induced to go to another person's home for a meal or even a friendly visit. I was just a boy then but was beginning to understand the term 'shut in'. One day, shortly after my return from the hospital to our home in the suburbs of Buffalo, New York, I made a solemn vow to bear my trial with a grin.

To that simple pledge, I owe my success in life not as a Champion Armless Golfer but just as a man who happens not to have any arms. Relating personal matters is not the easiest task, especially for me. However, I pray my story may give motivation to folks inclined to think they have insurmountable troubles and uncharitable burdens and they simply cannot play in the game of life anymore. And as strange as it may sound, I found in Golf life lessons unattainable anywhere else. An accurate picture of how this unlikely philosophy developed without returning to the year 1901 is impossible. Walter the fifth child to bless our family, arrived and being the oldest, it fell to me to play nursemaid and babysitter to the new infant. Oh joy! But there were rewards.

That year Buffalo New York played host to the Pan-American World Exposition of 1901 and my dad has his two-week vacation that year during the month of August. And since my Mom could not go, it was my good fortune to visit this once in a lifetime exposition with my father on almost a daily basis. Still fresh in my mind are those 14 days and the amazing technologies we saw. From a new radio called 'Stereo' to all-electric everything, to automatic new cars. It was easy to see that America had a bright future ahead, and I wanted my piece of that. I recall my dad buying me snacks of candy and peanuts and with my little hands I smeared the soft candy all over my face and clothes (one of the last recollections I have of using my hands).

Although only a tot, I recall the afternoon President McKinley was assassinated. Holding tightly to my father's powerful right arm, I was only 30 feet directly in front of the President when the fatal shot was fired. I was a witness to history on a very sad day for America, and it left an impression. The year 1901 showed me still with arms… but not for long.

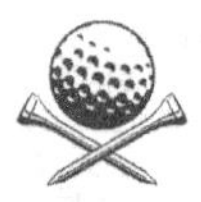

CHAPTER 4

Landing in the Rough
Suddenly Armless

"A leading difficulty with the average player is that he totally misunderstands what's meant by concentration. He's merely worrying."
Bobby Jones

September 13, 1901 was a beautiful crisp Fall day which will live with me forever. It was a day where the sky is bluer than blue; the leaves have started to turn and there's a cool bite to the air. We had only moved to the suburbs scarcely a month earlier. Although a little above our family budget, it was really in a great location right near the school, the hospital and perhaps most importantly, the Golf Course. Little did I understand that the God's well devised plan was laying a foundation for me.

That afternoon my Mother had gone to the city market. I was to help carry the food back to our house, so out into the afternoon sun I started up main street towards the market. I fell and before I knew it; the streetcar had taken both my arms. At the hospital the doctors were amazed I was still alive but they found it necessary to leave me armless just below the shoulder socket. I was not unconscious during the procedure, nope, not me, I chatted and joked with the Doctors and Nurses. I was on the operating table for 5 hours.

Think of it… armless. What an ugly handicap with which to start life. I thought my life was over. Perhaps most importantly, those I loved and respected also thought my life was over. In passing the fact that when the accident occurred and while in the hospital and to this very day I have never really had any pain, is marveled at by all who are familiar with what occurred that tragic day. As I look back upon the incident, it amazes me even to this day.

While in the hospital, my family brought me many delicious edibles every day; among other things were whole chickens, wine, candy, a variety of fruits, etc, Of course many of these things I was not allowed to eat but just looking at them was a pleasure. Everyone felt sorry for me and I hated it even though I'm sure they meant well but… My immediate family, Aunts, Uncles, Cousins and friends prayed that if it was "God's will" that I be taken in death. Can you imagine? Even though I was knocked out by drugs I could still hear them. But it was not His will because I'm still kicking about some 50 plus years later.

Mother, whenever she gets to feeling bad about my arms being gone, would always tell me "remember son, God left you here for a *reason*". A little egotistical, I know, but I still believe it to be true. The more I think about my Mother's admonition, the more I am convinced of her faith and that the

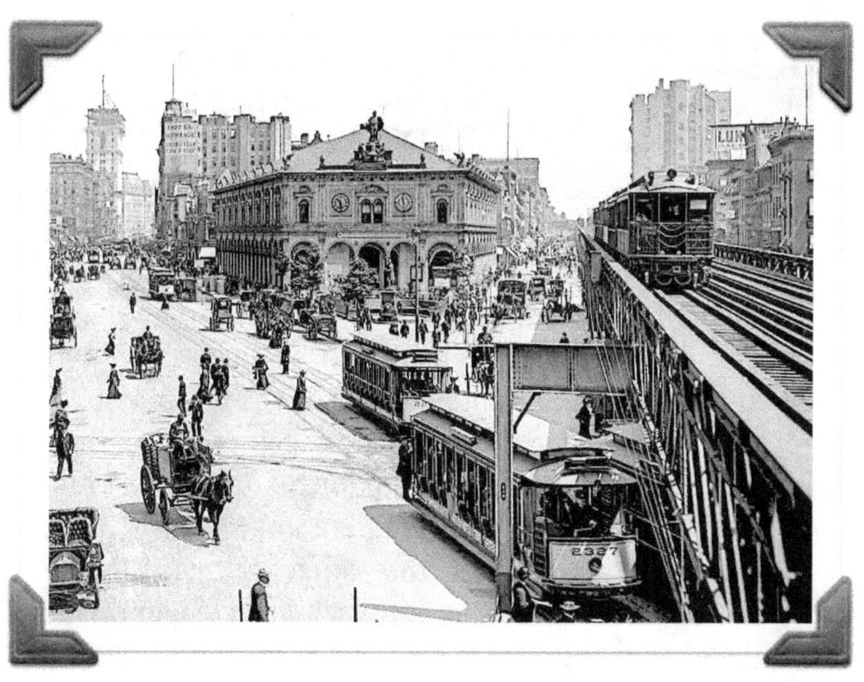

statement is true. As days come and go I trust God will use me for greater service to others.

During my convalescing days and really all through my life I've heard people say, "Gee Mac you sure were lucky the wheels didn't take your head off." Indeed I am grateful it didn't.

Naturally I could sit down on the sidelines put away the clubs and complain about the hand life had dealt me. I simply decided to love life despite the heartaches, sorrows and necessary hard knocks. It is sweet in all its aspects. As a youth I often wondered what "luck" had to do with my physical accident or with significant achievement. It was not until I had grown to manhood and had been kicked around plenty that I could finally fathom the word "luck".

And frankly, looking back, the accident was a blessing in disguise and I would not change a thing. Thousands of times I have heard friends and acquaintances say, "Gosh, I have had it tough and bad luck for all these years I sure wish a piece of good luck would fall my way!" This has been said in my presence so often that it's a mantra. Sadly, it creates an unnecessary handicap in every person's life as it is not fully understood. Luck, good or bad, to most folks way of thinking is something which happens to others and never happens to them. Most believe that it is fully out of our control. It's something which gives the other fellow all the breaks in life, in business and social circles, and was achieved with no effort on their part. Some people are just lucky. Did you ever stop and ask yourself why the other fellow has this so-called luck? Your friends were left a few million dollars, your best girl has gone to the Orient for a six months vacation, your pal in school who was considered a dunce has been been made head of a national concern… these things occur daily on all sides of us to others, but not to us of course.

You think there's nothing much you can do about it and hope that luck will climb your balcony. In fact you live with a hope that the curtains will part and the true luck feature picture will start. I've found that most folks are as happy as they make up their minds to be and that successful people make their own luck. The old George Burns adage "the harder I work, the luckier I get" comes to mind. And wishing avails you nothing. You can't name a single individual who became great just by wishing unless something more was added. Wishing is a beautiful dream however, we must couple it with thoughts and actions, not to mention tenacity. You must have the intestinal fortitude to consummate your wishing.

For years a man can plug away at his daily task and we see him as successful. Without warning, something happens, and they have made him head of his department or perhaps the company president. You and his friends might credit luck, however I would submit it's not. Luck or so-called luck does not materialize with one swing or one hole it directly results from numerous hits, many attempts and swing after swing after swing. After a while it puts you up on the green ready for a great putt. Each swing and each shot is a definite preparation for bigger and better things. We must crawl before wc can walk or run. We must have a straight and solid drive off the tee to be able to compete on the green. But it is our daily adherence to training and learning from our mistakes that the individual can then make his or her own luck.

One day your chance will come and when it does, even though it was hard work and effort and persistence, they'll still say you were lucky. The world is replete with examples. Just like when you're on the golf course doing those trick shots over and over or those 8 hour practice sessions, those efforts will give you the skills you need when you hit the rough and you're behind a big bush between you and the hole. So if you want luck in

your life, try these ideas:
1) Be prepared for when a break comes!
2) Stimulate your imagination and dream big!
3) Be you—you'll never get another chance!
4) Build your own luck with perseverance!

Not losing my head during the accident can't be called luck. It was a human body response and I choose to believe the will of God that I love. I trust as the years roll on that I will find it possible to teach this philosophy to the physically challenged and to every walk of life: the truth that there is no handicap in life except a mental one. Gee, where have I heard that before?

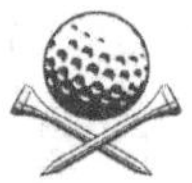

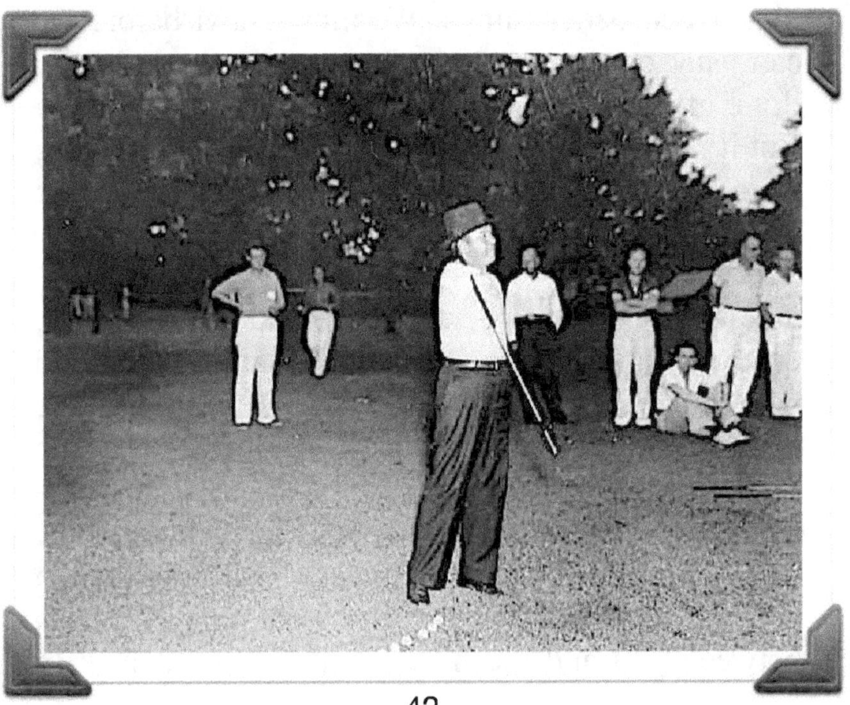

CHAPTER 5

Learning to be 'Handicapped'
Everything is Everything

"Concentration comes out of a combination of confidence… and hunger."
Arnold Palmer

"Even when times were good, I realized that my earning power as a golf professional depended on too many ifs and putts."
Gene Sarazen

Because I am armless and considered by millions of unthinking, unknowing people as helpless, I feel the need at this point of my humble story to give you a word picture on learning how to be physically handicapped. In living and proving the 'no handicaps' philosophy, I found out how vital it was to understand and embrace the art of being physically incapacitated. And there is an art and science to it. Caring for the physically imperfect in these United States has always been a problem since the birth of rehabilitation after the civil war. Today, with WWII vets, it is paramount both in practice and under the law that the issues of the disabled be addressed.

I limited this book to a general discussion because each case has unique characteristics that justly and merit individual rather than group consideration.

The daily battle to be positive is lifelong. And here's a Newsflash for some… probably immediate family members will prove of brief service in working it out, especially at the start. In most instances, members of the family insist upon saying things like "it's too bad " or "he'll be a burden the rest of his life." Of course, they may be well intentioned, however, no one can learn to be physically handicapped with such thoughts continually showered upon him or her. Upon the family's shoulders rest a specific duty, they can create about the individual an atmosphere of cheerful hopefulness with an abundance of dogged determination to help fill the gaps.

I have tried to allude to two groups; the first is the trained rehabilitation worker while the other is the experienced worker who is physically handicapped but who, previous to the defect, was a perfectly normal person. Further, one who has gone through the mill and is fully aware of the trials and tribulations facing the chap who is about to embark on his rehabilitation journey. It's difficult, but it can be done. The value of such a practitioner in teaching the imperfect how to live is unmeasurable.

In Golf we find the same thing in that one can learn the game much better by doing it than by reading about it. Further, I fully appreciate that every physically handicapped person is not qualified to fit into the same picture, but the best possible techniques should be utilized to the fullest extent possible. The reason is someone of this caliber usually inspires other handicapped humans and through concrete demonstrations of his capabilities and accomplishments. My Golf inspires others disabled and not alike. It helps them see that with the proper mental attitudes, proper training and guidance and a deep courage to carry-on that they too can succeed and live a fulfilling life. Aside from

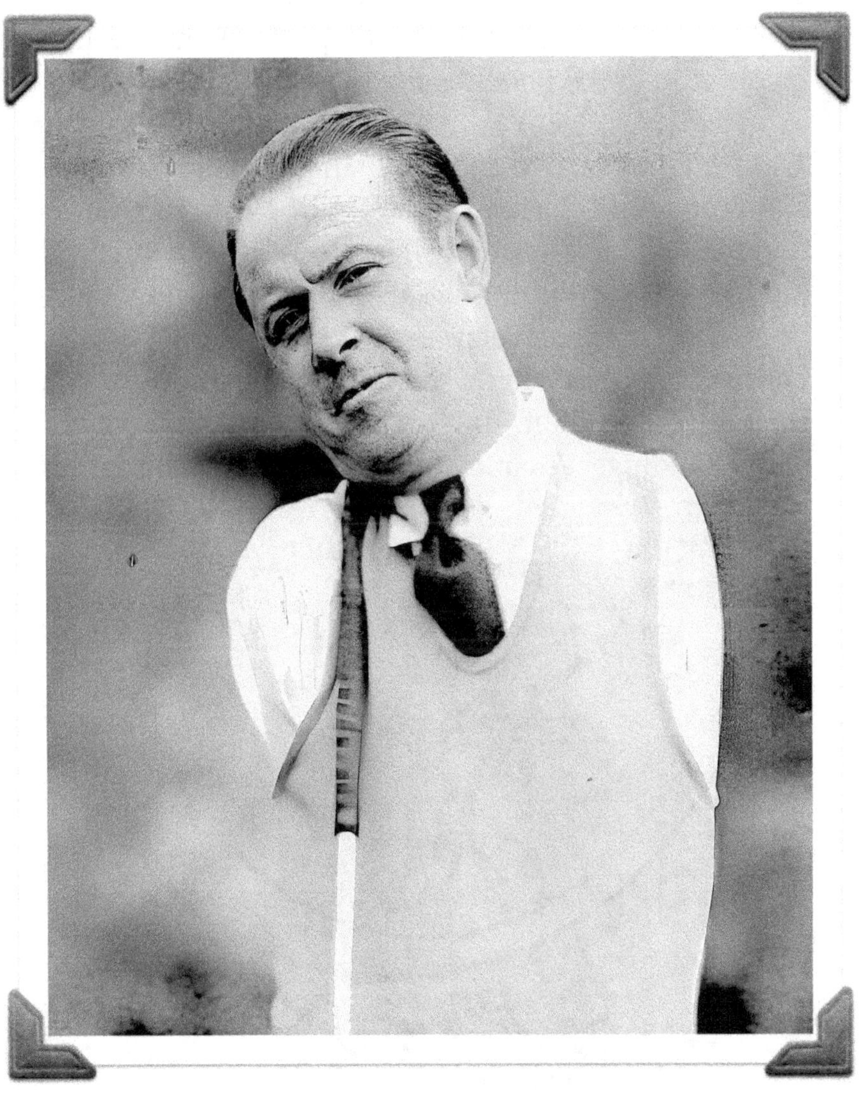

the ever apparent mental attitude so necessary for success, there's a physical problem confronting each individual. The problem is adjusting the individual to modern daily life and the act of doing things for self and a step-by-step retraining and regaining of self-confidence. It is the undeniable fact that a person blessed with the talents to help with this change plus an outstanding personality and a solid background to draw from will provide the needed inspiration in the patient's life.

We find physical disabilities in every community and among all classes of people in every section of our lives. The Physically handicapped are a small but integral part of our nation and as such, they must be studied in direct relation to our entire citizenship. Discussion of a single human problem is utterly impossible without first definitely establishing an understanding, a concrete relationship with other

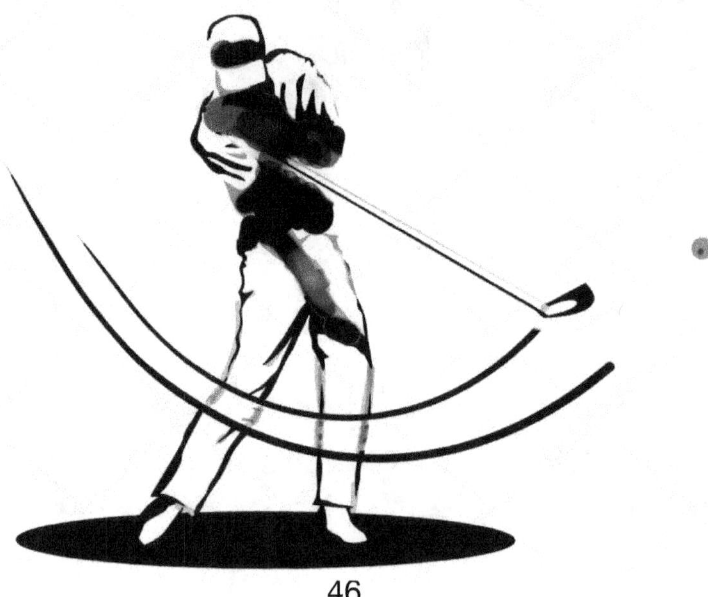

similar problems and how they interrelate. Our base must be one of perspective. You and I know only too well that derived values are but relative.

We also know that facts and truth of a half nature are far worse than unadulterated ignorance. Half-truths are always deceptive and prove very dangerous. The whole is only as strong as the weakest link. Accordingly, the real value is only securable by a concrete comparison with other human problems. In Golf, the handicap system of scoring was created so that player could measure themselves against one another and the sport on a fair and even basis. In rehabilitation, it's the results that count. You may have the ugliest swing in the world but if you get the ball in the hole that is all that really matters. For the afflicted, the measure is: can you live an independent life?

From experience, I state without fear of contradiction that learning how to be physically handicapped is easily the most difficult assignment of life. Such imposition clearly involves more than the restoration of a human soul. To me, any and all human souls are worthy and should be fully restored regardless of the trouble or cost. At first the horror and terror of an accident can be escaped or even lost sight of and maybe that's a good thing. From my experience when I first lost both arms, like thousands today upon whom physical impairment falls, one loses every sense of balance and proportion. That's exactly the way I felt at first but with a proper mental attitude adjustment, I have learned to feel and do things differently. Each individual immediately is encompassed with an obsession about their impairment, that this isolation, is only happening to them.

However, to overcome any handicap they must quickly learn the truth and see whole picture. They must be taught that they are a vital part of life and our communities. They are part of the web of life and must make the best of it and call in the full extent of their abilities. There's no need to repeat that when these conditions really exist in individuals, they actually believe hope for them is dead so it is time to remember those who have overcome the same challenges. What the other handicapped fellow can do is to emulate them. They're living proof that you can do as much and more with what you have if you'll make up your mind to do it. It is much easier said than done, my life in overcoming the hardship of losing both arms proves that learning to be physically challenged is *not* impossible.

Despite the challenges, I've been able to go through public high school and attend college. I write and operate a typewriter, feed myself, earn a good living and in fact I do just about everything for myself except dress and undressed. Luckily my wife helps! I have succeeded only because my mental attitude in life, my outlook, has been stubbornly positive. To back this up, I have made a strong finding that there really is no handicap in life except a mental one (where have I heard that before?). I see no reason why others can't do all that I have been able to accomplish and a lot more.

I consider the many wonderful things invented by Thomas Edison which have made our lives happier and more comfortable. Edison was deaf, but in accomplishing great inventions he proved handicaps could be overcome. He tried 1000 filaments before finding the right one and changing our world with the electric light bulb. Then there is the case of President Franklin D Roosevelt. He refused to let his physical defect deter him from serving others and fought hard to master his affliction with a clear-cut mental attitude backed by determination. He carried on and followed through despite his paralysis and had underlying faith in himself. This faith enabled him to reach the highest office in the United States and become one of our most beloved Presidents.

There are thousands upon thousands of shining examples of people throughout the world who have learned how to be physically challenged successfully. There is a lot to learn in this art of overcoming. Records show many individuals who before their physical impairment held positions of great responsibility and others who, through personal effort, built communities and great commercial enterprises. Having done these things, they had an abundance of business acumen which richly endowed them with education of the practical variety and a broader view on life. You might think that those experiences should enable each to accept their new condition in a more philosophical manner.

That's what should occur but it rarely does. In most instances these individuals fold it up in utter and complete despair. They will only withdraw, and that emotional response can be more debilitating than the injury itself.

Through personal experience I know this attitude to be unproductive and it should be discouraged. Just like in learning to be handicapped in Golf we learn and find our most authentic swing through repetition, the expertise of others and getting our mind to get out of the way of the body. The handicap challenge seems to be hopeful with people of the middle class. Those who are industrious and earning moderate wages also seem to better understand these concepts. This layer of our society, by being compelled to compete in the game of life for themselves, seem able to better grasp the no handicap concept. I'm not sure why.

Part of my early philosophy was to make the best use of those remaining physical factors I had. I wanted to regain my place in my community, state and nation. The question for me was how to make my physical remains do the things previously done. Well that and earn a decent living. This is a proper and perfectly natural question, and it's one that I am still grappling with to this day. A man has got to eat! I have been self rehabilitated and have been given more experiences in education than perhaps 90% of those in the handicapped community. It may sound odd, but I learned how to be physically handicapped. For those of you who have not learned this art yet

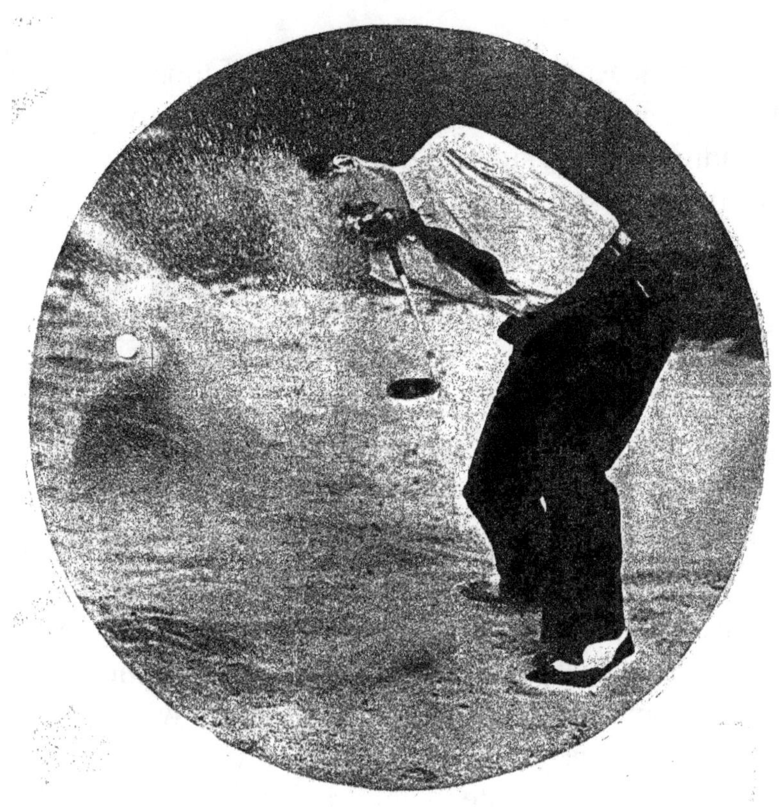

for your own self-preservation, you will need to face the problem squarely and it can sometimes not be beautiful. We still have to compete in the marketplace, only now we have an additional factor to deal with. But with a supportive environment, I'm in this competition to win and that belief can make all the difference.

The factors of motivation, perseverance, competition are vital in life. With an accident such as mine, all these ambitions and personal hope for the future has been blasted away. Not through any wild stretch of the imagination can such individuals be consoled or made to believe that life's future holds anything for them, at least at first. It is almost as if those affected have stepped out of line and are seemingly just standing by the side of the road. Yes, standing and waiting for someone to pick them up. All effort to cheer or consoled is simply wasted energy. Nevertheless, he must not be left standing there, no matter how disgruntled or combative he might be or become. We must make such individuals to see the light through the eyes of an individual who has accomplished things under a physical handicap.

The person carrying a physical burden should, at the very beginning, emulate the doings of other successful handicapped people. Have them mimic, for a while a successful person who has learned how to be handicapped and their courage will return. Emulating the doings of successful handicapped people has far greater encouraging power than the direction by those who have studied the problem. Having someone analyze your swing and tell you what is wrong is not nearly as effective as them showing you what is amiss. The problem's individualized and no one size fits all. We learn best by doing and that's true in rehabilitation and in Golf.

As previously stated the problem is not an individual one. How long will the individual remain standing by the roadside? That depends much upon themselves. How long will they allow a slice to ruin their game? Same thing. I often marvel at how some Golfers will spend big money on clubs and outfits and all the accessories, yet not a dime for lessons to learn how to be a better player. Hope and perseverance are essential in overcoming any handicap, but like luck they must come from within and must be put into action by the individual. A good mental attitude is vital to success in overcoming a handicap and in the game of Golf. Encouragement and empathy, but under no circumstance sympathy, is paramount to each person overcoming physical imperfections.

The proper outlook on life's future and the proper mental attitude will materialize when the physical imperfect folks realize, of their own volition, that they're not the only physically incapacitated humans in the world. Until each individual fully realizes this they are bound to experience many heartaches and depressing moments. and feelings of isolation, but once they realize they are not alone nor handicapped and are provided with the proper stimulus to go forward they will do so.

When Golfers find out that others have the same or a similar slice or defect, they both feel better and are motivated to make the changes needed to improve their game. My progress at the beginning was rather slow but on the other hand as I have stated before, the handicapped individual and the physician who is associated with them, have "gone through the mill of experience" and have succeeded sometimes in spite of themselves. By associating with a handicapped chap who has scaled the heights, he will be encouraged and will clearly feel the urge of ambition quickly regaining his lost self-confidence. As a further result his motto gradually but surely will become "I can do anything the other fellow can do," and when that glimmer in the eye returns it is indeed something to see. Through personal experience in learning how to be physically handicapped as well as my years on the lecture platform and over the airwaves, I'm positive the most valuable factors for the physically handicapped are personal and one on one associations.

Progress will be facilitated if the individual, once he knows his physical condition can't be further improved, consoles himself to that fact and determines that during the years which lay ahead he will tackle the limitations with every ounce of intelligence and strength in his being. Once having gained a solid attitude towards self and life, there is another factor the disabled must know. It's simply life's attitude towards us (it does not care) and how mindset is solely of his own making. I have often counseled that a smile is an asset no man can afford to be without. Smile and the world smiles with you but weep and you will cry alone. This truism applies to the everyone.

Personally? I ask no quarter from life or my fellow man except fair-play and equal opportunities. A physical handicap does not mean oblivion in business in social life athletics or life itself... the physical loss does not mean or even imply a loss of mental abilities. Those who do something for the physically handicapped, helping them help themselves, let this be first last and always: "Let us first seek to inspire, and do our teaching after our inspiration has been firmly rooted in others". Having learned how to be physically handicapped successfully, I've tried throughout my life and in this book to put down those factors and human characteristics which have helped me in overcoming the loss of my two arms. Those 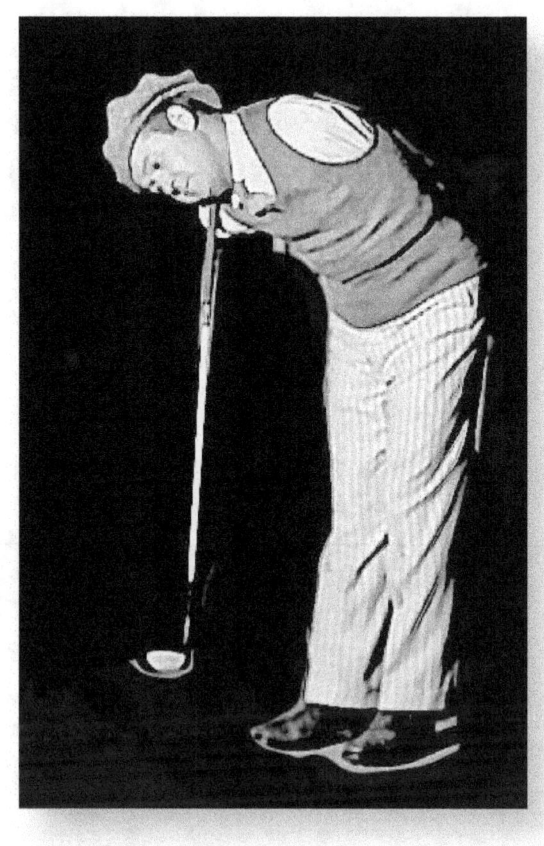 factors which have assisted me are easily duplicatable. Dear reader, I lay no claim to being the best writer. I have not attempted to be an academic, just offer my philosophy to anyone one who is interested..

It is my humble and sincere hope that the reader will derive some comfort, some education and a keener interest in self and how the game of Golf can help create a deeper interest in both his internal self and his fellow man regardless of their condition. If just one individual who reads this is prompted in courage to do something for himself or another, my reward will be ample and my mission complete. There were those throughout my life, well-meaning though they were, who said I should not even try, that I would never be able to actually play a round of Golf. That I should just live on charity the rest of my life and let others do for me and watch other folks play Golf... Fat chance!

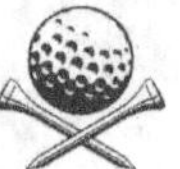

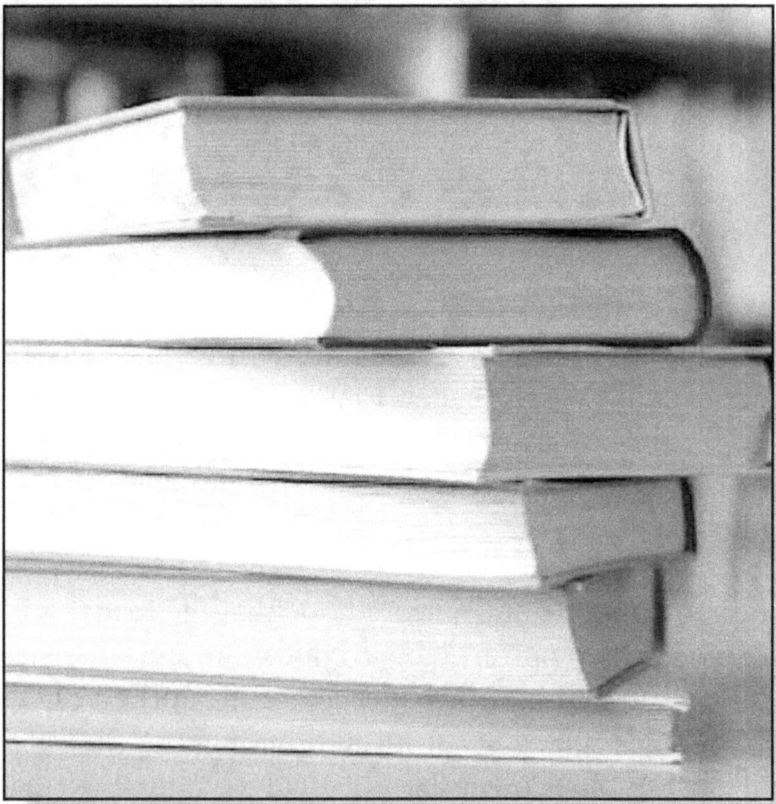

CHAPTER 6

An Education
The Great Equalizer?

"Golf is not a game of good shots. It's a game of bad shots." Ben Hogan "In golf as in life, it is the follow through that makes all the difference."
Anonymous

After 13 days in the hospital they sent me home (and you wonder why 13 is my lucky number?) The fall school term was well underway when I returned from the county hospital. My heart ached as I saw the other kids in my neighborhood with books and slates tucked under their arms scampering off to school. After school I watched them through my window, with tear filled eyes as they played in the afternoon sun.

There I was, armless, and as tears trickled down my cheeks I finally realized that I could not play ball, climb trees or shoot a slingshot as my playmates were doing in the fields just across the street. It was a tough but necessary realization. I returned to school the last of October with the determination that nothing would deter me from completing the long arduous journey to some sort of successful career via education.

For immigrant Irish education was the great equalizer and even at an early age I understood this.

Naturally like most young men, I dreamed of being a pro baseball player or professional Golfer on the PGA tour. It's a sad hard truth when you come to realize you won't achieve your dreams. So if then it becomes time to go find new dreams. After a few years of learning how to learn then came graduation year and "Little Tommy" gathered his second victory when I was elected President of my Senior Class. People seemed to like me and I was making progress. I was also Caddying and fooling around with my discarded Golf club. And perhaps most importantly, I was doing things for myself although I was still very sensitive about my limitations.

Realizing my future depended in large part upon education, I entered central high school. I now fully understood that I must make up in brain power what I lacked in arm power. By this time I could conduct myself in the classroom as efficiently as any other

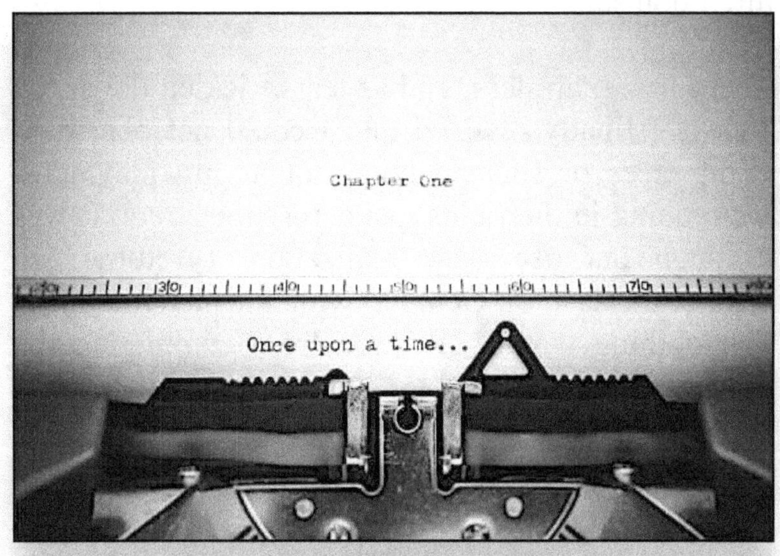

normal student. Here's the picture… I could write and was able to "handle" papers, books, a ruler, a compass with neatness and dispatch by utilizing my lips and teeth as fingers. Once the novelty wore off they left alone me to learn. And that's exactly what I did. Athletics had always caught my fancy. In fact before the arm amputation, I was determined in my mind that I was going to make my mark in sports.

If I could not play I could still take part and in high school I received exceptional honors by being selected Team Manager of both the Football and Baseball teams for two consecutive years. Running was also a favorite past time of mine. I gained the habit by running to the golf club and around the golf course every day after school. I was also a member of my school relay team so this was good training. And we did well in track meets around the area. While still in high school I competed in a marathon race of about 12 miles and for some reason still unknown to me I was clocked in as the 13th runner to cross the tape.

But the thing I'm still most proud of is the fact that I started and finished the race. From high school I matriculated at Michigan State University in Lansing Michigan and there I specialized in animal husbandry. I had fancied myself a future farmer… Can you picture an armless farmer? I could. Strange as it seems I have never followed my vocation except informally. I started out to be a scientific farmer, but wound up being a positive thinking Golfer instead. Sadly, I had to leave college at the end of my freshman year not because I did not like school or wasn't doing well but simply because my family could not afford to keep me there.

Regrets? Friends, I have none. I think perhaps the most important lesson I learned while at college was in fact how to learn. How to go to a public library and research subjects of interest, that was the key that unlocked the door to independent knowledge for me. Nowadays my vocation is working for and in the interest of the world's greatest fraternity—-the physically challenged. I delight in doing something for the other fellow, and above all helping the afflicted help themselves. To me, no greater service is possible.

Now I understand that advice is dirt cheap and over the years I have received more than my fair share. I am also fully appreciative of the fact that success requires courage by the physically strong, and a double dose of courage for the physically afflicted. For us to battle life successfully, it must be all hands on deck at all times.

When I hear of some robust individual with every physical advantage say "I wish I was dead," I would delight in shaking him until he was blue in the face! That's if I had two hands, of course... This unhealthy remark means but one thing... that the individual has no reason for living only because they have lost their "courage" to go on and live life fully. With the 'no handicaps' mindset, it's necessary to have a wealth of deeply rooted courage to draw

upon, not just to overcome the physical imperfections, but also a daily beat down from all the prevalent prejudice against handicapped individuals. As a matter of fact you have many potent reasons for living but it's up to you to find them. No one will do it for you. Like Golf such lessons are simple not easy.
'

My life experience in proving 'no handicaps' shows that positive thought is less prevalent among the physically challenged than the average person in America today. A lack of courage mixed with a good dose of self-pity is a concoction for failure. God gave life for us to use and we can stay in ignorance, fear and resentment without courage or we can simply get on with it. I know it's easier said than done but what other choice is there? Just imagine life supplying you with reasons for living.

Franky, it's your job and yours alone, to furnish your own reasons for living. When you hit the Links the same applies; it's up to you to use your clubs and find your best way to the hole and no two routes to the flag are the same. It may sound harsh but the sooner you realize it the better. The way to courage may be simple but it is surely difficult.

I am fully aware of the problems facing the physically challenged as well as normal folks during these trying times. So we must ask, when is a man a failure? I would submit it's when he is no longer willing to try. But what is success? I would share with you that my definition of success drastically

A Cultivating Swing

*Such a clever lad. Quicker than a shadow. Oh his ability to
put the small white ball in the little hole was par for all to
see. All the gang said he's our honey and they backed him
with their money. When the ball rolled not his way they
couldn't seem to get him down to the wonder of the Butch.
The other fellows knew it, they thought he couldn't do it. He
grinned and thought life so fancy and
found a swing calm and quiet.*

*Let the fancy swingers run riot. He found the chance he
needed and landed on the green and on the mat they're lying
reposing, found a winning team. They held the man a winner,
he's got a swing punch but there was nothing new about his
story no it's just an allegory. There is a moral think it over,
it's a tip and there are a bunch.*

*Life's an 18 hole round and in case you want to do it and
win it, cultivate your swing!*

By Tommy McAuliffe
Poem written in 1936

changed on that crisp fall day when the street car rode away with both my arms. In my humble opinion, a person who is en route to being a failure is one who lacks or has completely lost his courage. Without courage, life is hopeless. And if you are to overcome any limitation, physical or mental, you will need a good dose of courage…

At birth, with brains capable of doing the seemingly impossible with or without a strong body, we're all equipped with all the tools needed to win. Remembering as you must that there is no handicap in life except in one's own mind, with your formidable asset, your brains, it's up to you to find your own courage and reasons to move forward. After a flying start which gives every promise of going on forever, you receive a setback, a good sock on the chin. You falter, you quit, you refuse to play further. You are simply afraid to go on and you've become weaker. How silly! Do you think life will politely rap at your door, enter your house, pat you on the back and pick you up from the blow which just felled you? Not a chance. I've waited and waited and waited and the knock never comes.

That's exactly what life does not do. Life is time and time is the only aviator that flies with safety. Life goes on in its definite way and never sidetracks itself for you nor anyone. Life allows you to play the ball exactly where it lay and it's up to you to find your best stroke to get to the green. Got knocked down? Get up or take the consequences. Opportunity has been afforded to each of us but if you don't care to play the game of life with all the rules in force, it's simply not the fault of life. You alone, are the loser and all because you lack "courage." What a waste!

This abstract idea of courage became my dominant force in overcoming the loss of my two arms. It was simple courage for me and can be courage for you. Through personal experience I found there's no better stimulant for reversing a complete loss of courage than to study the lives of distinguished men and women who have carried on through thick or thin to great heights. The same is equally true of physically complete individuals who started life under adverse circumstances and who, with courage and effort, reached the top of the ladder of their respective fields, but perhaps more importantly, became successful in life. Look about you and you will uncover thousands of people who are worth studying. What tools and techniques do they use to be successful and how can those tools be adapted to your life? When matters look hopeless, when you think you would like to just give up and end it all, that's the time you must do something for yourself.

Here's a technique I have found very helpful. Gather under your arm a bunch of pictures of "greats" who have thrived under handicaps and have succeeded in life. Then go quickly to your room and there hold an Open Meeting. Set the pictures about the room and contemplate each of them. What made them great? I am positive in the company of these greats your courage will return. In that bundle of pictures is a person whose courage to overcome his physical handicap allowed him to become President of the United States. Yep Franklin Delano Roosevelt.

Going deeper into the pile you'll uncover a snapshot of Helen Keller… Deaf, dumb and blind from birth she has done great things, greater perhaps than you and I will ever do with our normal faculties. She helped the blind to see, the deaf to hear and the mute to speak. Another example would be that of a tall thin Jewish man pushing a saw in a carpenters shop… Jesus of Nazareth… from whose simple life sprang the greatest religion in the history of mankind. Not bad for a Jewish Carpenter.

Among the images is also a picture of a tall skinny man outside a humble log cabin. With 17 attempts to gain public office he was a failure yet Abraham Lincoln became President and saved our nation from Civil War. Near the bottom of the pile of pictures you may be holding a portrait of Dr. Benjamin Franklin who walked the streets with bread laden pockets as the people laughed at him,

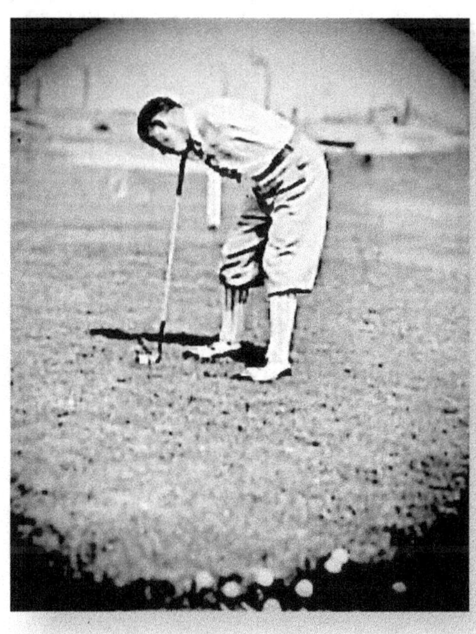

yet he helped create our country and significantly contributed to science. If you have lost your courage or if you have not a full measure of it, study these pictures and read the life stories of eminent men and women.

When this has been done, rush to a mirror and as you gaze at its smooth shiny reflective surface… Smile. Unfolded to your eye and your subconscious mind is the fact that you are no worse than Roosevelt, Keller, Christ, Lincoln or Franklin. Through courage they surmounted a great handicap and if they can so can you.

My successes despite having no arms are quite simply because of courage which willingly says "I can do it" and "I will do it". Never taking no for an answer and realizing that without courage no man can even hope to really succeed. And by the way that courage need not be and often isn't necessarily heroic. Often we may wonder why others pass us by in life. There are chaps who have become headliners yet have less talent than others. How do you account for it? And there's fear of endeavor leaving you behind. How do you account for it? What mystery power possesses them? How are they particularly brilliant? In the final analysis their achievements were possible only through persistent effort. When a tough job presented itself they tackled it and did it. What do you do? Perhaps you back away saying "Gee I can't do it." The other fellow had courage enough to go out on the sales call or play the match while you stayed at home. Who won? He has at least the courage to try.

Often you have a song in your heart but you won't sing it because no one else is singing? The Teacher asked you to talk to the group or class gathering but you refused because you were afraid of making a mistake or saying the wrong thing? The other person did it and she is now the group leader. They had courage while you lacked it. After suffering a big bundle of hard knocks, it may finally dawn upon you that life is not to blame, it is you who are because you have been lacking in courage, initiative, knowledge or whatever. It indeed can be a sad awakening. It's up to you if you want to live, and if you want to live fully.

Do you want to be up on the Tee ready to play or do you want to be just another watcher in the Gallery? Courage will do it. With courage there would be no chronic whiners or quitters. Therefore if you would be part of life, if you would be an asset to yourself, if you would be an asset to your community, state and nation. If you would be of service to society, and if you would be a real man or woman for your family, you must find your courage however you personally define it. It is courage which has moved mountains and it was courage which enabled prominent men and women to arrive at the top of the mountain.

It will be the same courage which will either stamp you as a figure to be entered in red, meaning failure,

on the ledger of life, or in black, meaning success, as the years roll by. How much courage? I do not know, I only know that without it, proving 'no handicaps' would have been simply impossible. Courage, however you find it, is vital to overcoming life's obstacles and in providing a total
education for life.

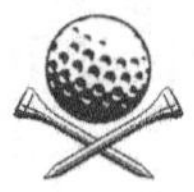

CHAPTER 7

Learning to Do the Impossible
Repetition Towards Perfection

"To the timid, everything is impossible."
Sir Walter Scott

My service and underlying interest in the work of improving the lives of the physically handicapped is only exceeded by my interest and activity in the sport of Golf. It was the 1930s and Golf was more popular than ever. It was my new field of dreams. I had caddied during my newspaper delivery days and I had watched golfers at my local golf course thru the fence. Yeah, but how? I would ask myself. Think of it, an armless man trying to play the most exasperating game in the world. I thought about it and watched others do it for a long time. To be close to the game, I began carrying the clubs of others as often as I could. And over time, I learned not just the mechanics of the game, but the etiquette and sportsmanship as well.

My progress at Golf was slow at first, but it was not long until I had the gumption to compete in the annual Caddy Golf Championship for the beautiful prizes donated by club members. Competition was fierce, but it was my good fortune to win this championship on two occasions in 1911 and 1912. My game advanced to the point where I was able to negotiate the difficult Country Club 18 holes in only

108 strokes. Par was 72. This is a not a remarkable score as scores go, but it made me very proud. I was doing the seemingly impossible and it felt good. Only about 80% of golfers with both arms are capable of playing 18 holes in only 108 strokes. I was only 15 when my first par score was made and recorded. From 1932 until 1933 I played 262 rounds of Golf on almost as many golf courses and had an average score per round of 92. '

'To date as I write this I have traveled nearly 1,000,000 miles playing the wonderful game of golf. And in the past few years I have hit a golf ball approximately 319,000 times. I can tell you without hesitation that the lessons learned later in life are the same ones I learned early on at the golf course. In 1920 when the local district Golf Association was formed I was elected its Secretary and served in that capacity for nine years. While serving as Golf Secretary I was also attached to the Buffalo News as its Golf Reporter/Editor and it was my yearly pleasure to cover the National Championships.

Those assignments will forever be cherished by me and as I look back upon them it was a sound schooling of the practical kind from the best strikers on the planet. The 13 1/2 years covering golf in the media were golden. Through reporting on golf I have met most of the golf greats including Bobby Jones from Atlanta, Walter Hagan from Detroit, Jim Dowdy from Los Angeles and trick shot golfer Joe Kirkwood from New York, just to name a few.

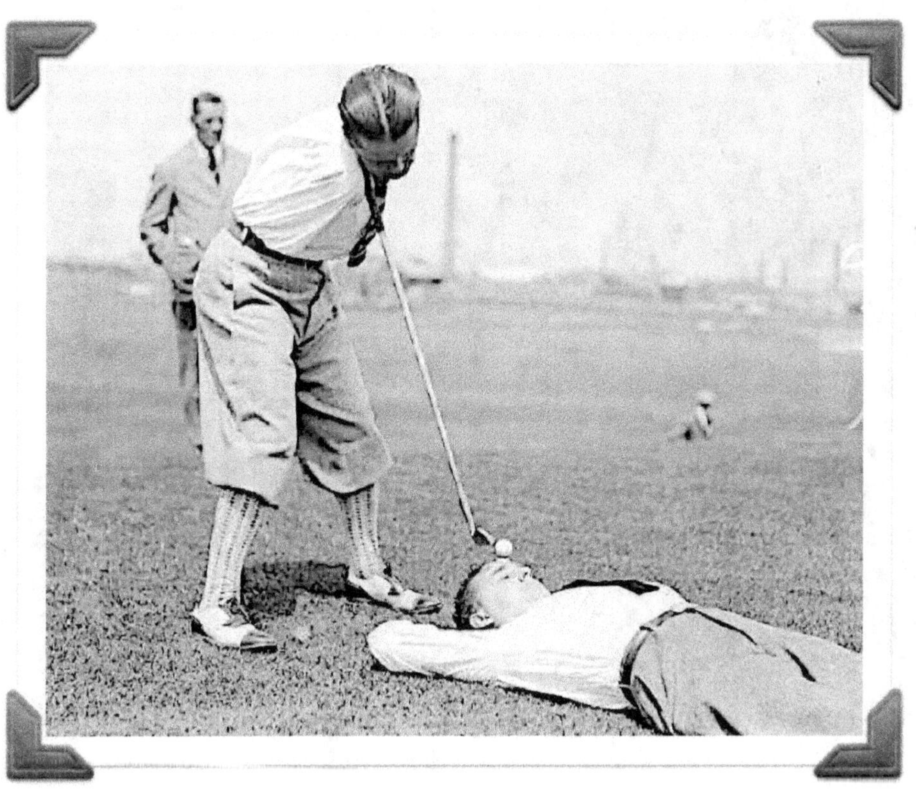

The Author's Dad, Bob, tests out Tommy's concentration

As a Golfer I have displayed my swing in every state in the United States, every province in Canada and every territory of Australia. I have been captioned "America's foremost trick shot Golf expert." As part of my indoor and outdoor exhibitions, I drive a ball from the crystal of a watch and then I go myself one better by driving a ball off a human forehead. In both instances I use only a candy Lifesaver to separate the ball from the watch or fore head. Folks love it. The only explanation for never having broken a watch crystal or skin on a forehead is my power of concentration.

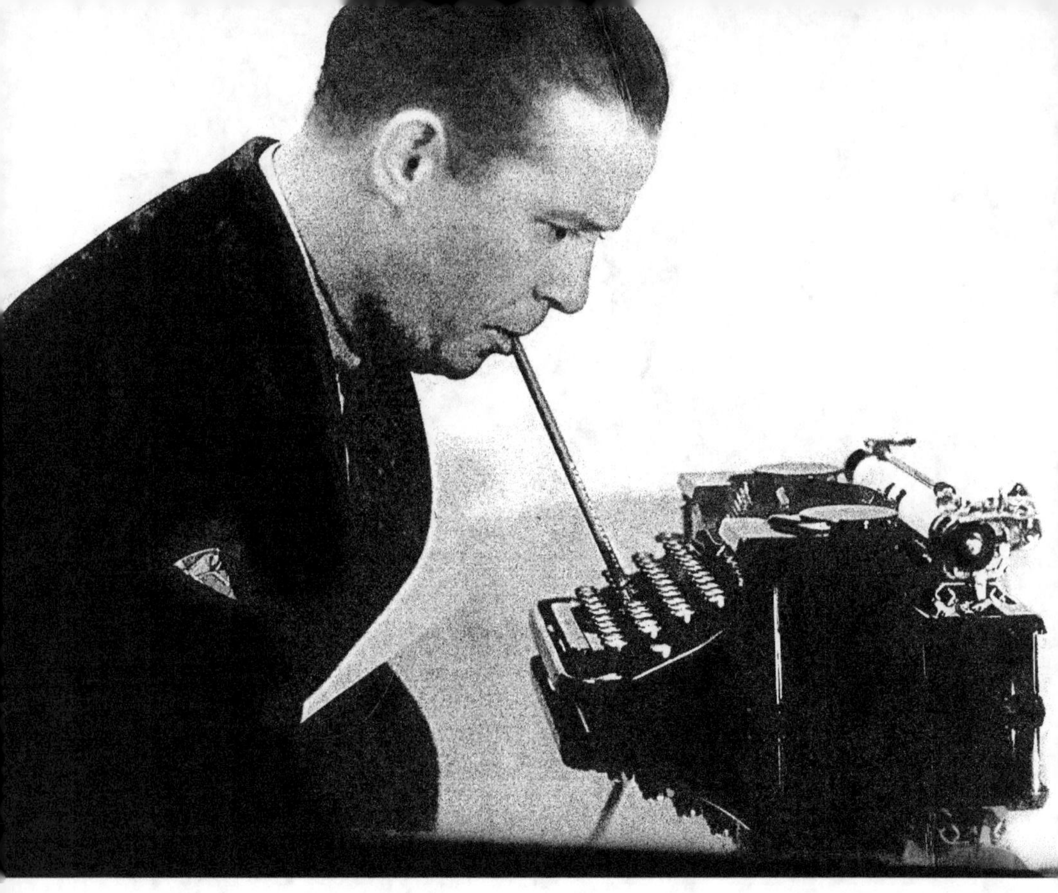

This power has been a major factor in producing measurable repeatable results in both my life and my golf game. Over the years my game has improved by 16 strokes and I attribute this improvement in large part due to my mental discipline in the game. For the curious my clubs are ordinary; the length is 42 1/2 inches, the Woods weigh 16 ounces and the Irons, 15 ounces. I carry 17 clubs, Bobby Jones 'Model 13' Irons and four Woods. Believe it or not I use every club to good advantage during a full 18 holes. Par is my best score to date. I've made PAR four times. Not bad for a guy with no arms!

With my Drivers, my distance is about 150 to 200 yards. Not long but at least they are straight! With

Irons, the yardage is about 100-125 yards. What I lack in distance I make up for in accuracy on the fairway. I hit straight golf balls! I attribute my ability to score so well in being able to control my short game on the Green and my keen putting eye.

According to OB Keller, who writes for the Atlanta Journal Newspaper and is considered by many to be America's greatest Golf Writer, I am some Golfer. Back in 1932 he wrote this in the Atlanta Journal:

"Tommy McAuliffe is as much a genius with woods, irons and putters as the renowned Golfer Bobby Jones!" I am honored and have developed a fast friendship with the golfing great Olympian. To be a journalist, operating a typewriter is essential. I learned to do this as a youth and later as a Reporter. Holding a pen or pencil in my mouth I wrote every word of this book on my typewriter letter by letter. Not once but six times! I solve the seemingly impossible problem by using an ordinary pencil with a large eraser on one end with which the keys are hit and the carriage moved. The other end is held between my lips and teeth. I actually type about 35 words per minute on one of my 3 Royal typewriters.

In my travels around the world I have had many interesting interviews and it was while playing the Paramount Theater in New York City that I was interviewed by Philadelphia Ledger and NBC Radio. I explained that I did not consider myself to be special, I merely refuse to be defeated by the loss of a couple of arms. I use what God has left me, my

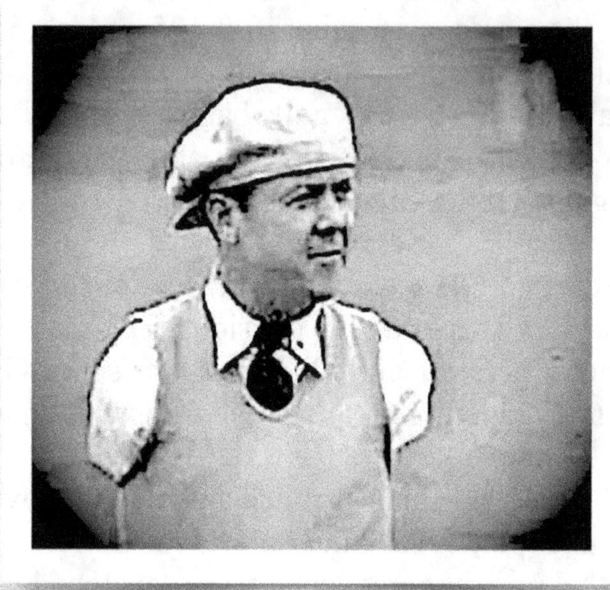

brains and my two good legs. In proving I had no handicaps I found that the battle is usually within. In learning to do the impossible… Playing Golf or operating a Typewriter… I believe I have partially proven the "no handicap" philosophy. When they amputated my arms just below the shoulder, luckily they didn't amputate my brain.

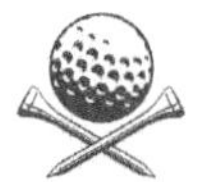

CHAPTER 8

If it's meant to be… it's up to me!
Nobody is Coming to help

"The only time my prayers are never answered is on the golf course."
Billy Graham

"Man cannot discover new oceans unless he has the courage to lose sight of the shore."
Andre Gide

I have come to believe that it's if gonna be, it's up to me. To be a 'somebody', to be a success, whatever that is to you, is an innate trait in the breast of every human being. No one will dispute that perseverance plus confidence were the factors that made the difference in my life. The present and future will not only require but demand a greater abundance of perseverance and confidence if you want to make it in this modern world. Talk is cheap my friend, and as free as the air we breathe.

It's not my intention to be preachy but offer a honest assessment, talking heart to heart with you. Thoughts are funny things and must be controlled and practiced daily in the ultimate hope of becoming a better person, a better man, a better Father, a better Husband not to mention a better Golfer.

The two other essential elements, perseverance and confidence, while they are two different and distinct words and attributes, they are so closely related I feel the need to link them together. Let me give you a sentence picture of the two words as taken from the dictionary: Perseverance -to keep on by force of will despite discouragement and obstacles. Confidence- Your state of mind which is characterized by reliance upon yourself regardless of your environmental circumstances or physical challenges. Simple addition and we get a picture of these combined words which in my mind mean this: going forward despite physical imperfections and with full and complete confidence in your own ability to rise to the top of your coveted objective.

I have no doubt that every reader of 'No Handicaps' listened to the blow-by-blow description of the Max Baer and James Braddock heavyweight fight in the Summer of 1934. It was one of the most listened to broadcasts in history. This fight carries a real story... A timely moral for every man and woman living today. Braddock won because he proved to be a better fighter. However the reasons go further and deeper. It was indeed a perfect example of perseverance and confidence.

In 1932 Braddock was considered a "has been" and counted out by the boxing press as well as by the public. But he had different ideas about it. He continued in his own way to carry on because in his own mind he had confidence in his ability to go forward and reach the goal of the Title. He said often both publicly and I'm sure to himself, "I can win and I will win" this was confidence in himself in spite of the contrary thoughts of the world. He backed this confidence trait with unshaken perseverance to carry on and follow through regardless of obstacles in his path or the opinions of others.

Braddock's reward for self-confidence and perseverance was to be rewarded with the World Heavyweight Title. With confidence backed by consistent repetition you can be a somebody in your chosen vocation. I have found human failures are not the result of physical imperfections nor the incompleteness of knowledge nor the lack of money.

Friends, human failures result from the absence of a proper mental attitude and the perseverance to keep hitting the ball. Perseverance is a medicine and life tonic. Its recipe is equal parts courage and confidence. It is only right that you ask yourself "what volume of confidence and perseverance do I have?" I'll never be convinced that it's a hopeless physical condition which creates a handicap. There are any number of physically imperfect humans known to you who readily disapprove such thinking. To me a handicapped person is simply created through another utter lack of mental application. It's this lack of mental fiber which impedes your forward growth. It will deprived you of the opportunity of reaching your goals.

One must realize the simple truth that having ideas and ambitions alone will not materialize your desires. The unemployment office is filled with folks who had great ideas but never acted upon them. Unless these dreams are vigorously acted upon you have wasted your energy. Remember the following and it will serve you well: having confidence in yourself and your ideas is the initial essential tool to undertaking things which are great. When the curtains close don't give anyone a chance to say about you "his life was wasted doing nothing". People who do nothing are usually crippled in their spirit, as my Mom use to say. It is a much more deadly affliction.

With confidence in your own ability to do big and worthwhile things backed by your unyielding perseverance to keep your eye on the ball, it will simply be impossible for you to be crippled in spirit and you will ultimately succeed. In reaching your goals many obstacles will block your path. Laziness is but one obstacle which will give you plenty of trouble and unless you can kick it into the trashcan of life, you will usually be deprived of victory. To be lazy is usually to admit that you lack confidence in yourself, sometimes a low energy level is a medical problem that should be looked at. And of course without our new found confidence you will be void of perseverance. Laziness is also a deadly form of doubt. 'Why bother, I know I can't do it.'

And as I'm sure you realize, you won't be reaching your goals without plenty of hard work. Don't be a loafer or unproductive member of your family or community. Your life success, your happiness,

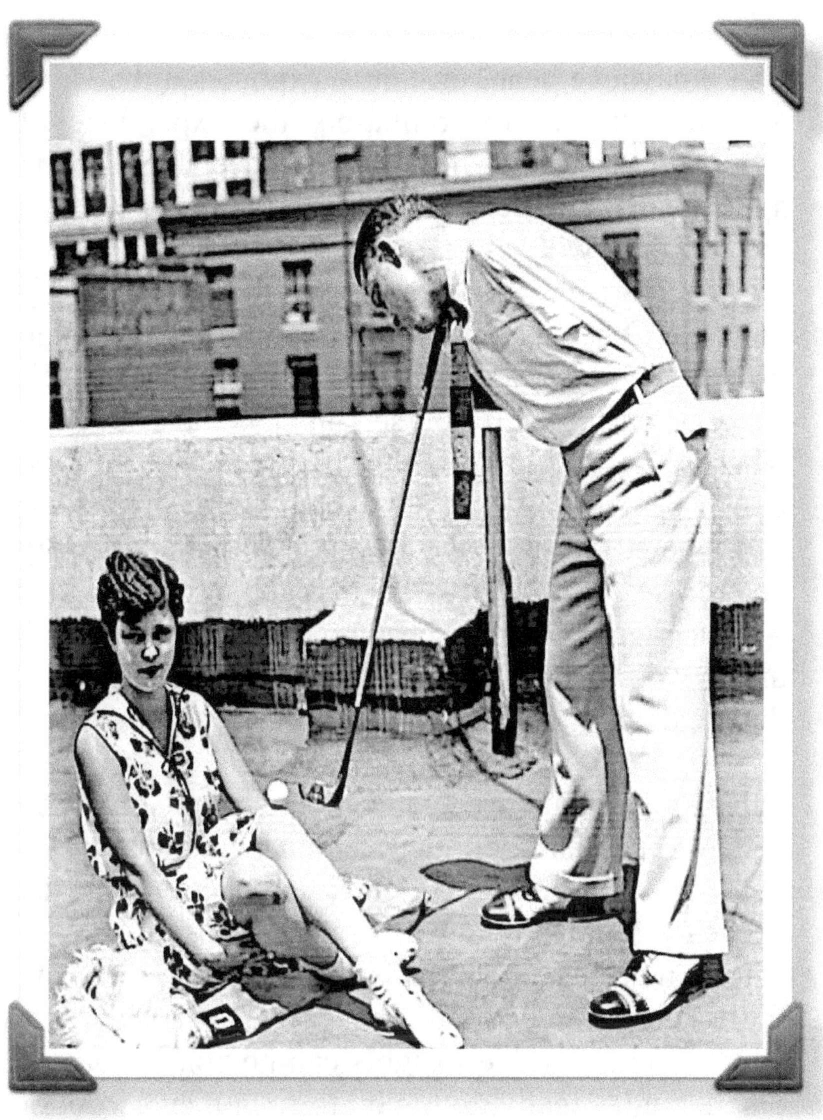

Rooftop Exhibition, Los Angles, CA 1940

depends entirely upon your being active as well as productive. Ten years from now when you view your life in retrospect, will you be able to say in all fairness to others and yourself that you have accomplished something? Something true and unique? You can, but it's up to you and you alone.

These days we hear constantly expounded the value and necessity of rehabilitation, the experience of special schools and the need for special prosthetic appliances. I appreciate how important each of these are but they will prove of no benefit to you unless you decide right here now to do things in helping yourself. Others can point the way, but it's up to you to make your life a success or failure. Which will it be? Out on the Golf course I always have to smile when some new player hits the links with all new clubs, bag, shoes (and God help us even a color coordinated outfit!), and he hits the ball miserably yet refuses to take lessons and then some Duffer with a raggedy set of beat up Irons and shoots 3 under Par. Was it because of the Clubs? Or was it a thing called practice?

Other individuals or organizations cannot give you perseverance and confidence, only you can, and as with anything else you must practice the skills needed. Your individual situation will ultimately determine these necessary life factors for you. Experience in my own life has proven to me that the way to these coveted insights can be pointed out by others but it's really up to you to find, then accept or reject them. Rejecting them spells defeat and accepting them is the pathway to winning. It's really that simple.

This medicine works for every individual regardless of race, religion, political affiliation, physical condition or previous condition of life, but only if we are willing to put in the work. I pray you were already gifted with confidence and perseverance. Should you be short on these, do not expect to make them yours overnight. You must be patient. You must grow with them from day to day. Remember, patience is a virtue worth cultivating. Perhaps you have confidence and are decided in your own mind to persevere on your path, then suddenly you make a mistake. One mistake will matter very little if you don't stop there. When such events happen to you remember this, just because you failed once, twice or 1 million times you don't want to be termed a failure until you are dead or you have lost your confidence and perseverance and quit. I always remember that Thomas Edison tried more than 1000 different filaments before he found the right one and created the electric lightbulb changing our world. What if he had stopped at 999?

The brave are always the favorites in life's great race. Long ago it was said, "God hates a coward." As I see it, the best way to achieve confidence and perseverance is a definite attack. A plan of battle. By being prepared to meet the obstacles which life hands you, you'll be well prepared if you have confidence and perseverance. I decided the necessary step to this is looking on the bright side of things. It's your attitude. You have sense enough to know that come what may, nothing is so bad that it could not be worse. We would be well to not gloom and doom and worry our way to the cup and but rather never doubt our own ability to reach Par. Maybe you can't hit a hole in one. So what? At least you're on the course of life playing the game. Enjoy it! Don't construe my thoughts to mean that life is all fun and games.

It's not, in any stretch of the imagination. I would not have you believe for a second that it's not essential to take your life seriously. It is vital that you constantly think and firmly believe that things are not as bad as they seem and that tomorrow will render better things for you. When you are able to do this you will have won at least half of your life's battles. You must add to this a firm belief that you have a definite place in life's full scheme of things. And this realization, regardless of your imperfections, can go a long way towards personal peace. You are where God intended you to be. It may sound a little shopworn but believe it or not you are the undisputed captain of your life's ship. Accordingly it's up to you to chart your life's course through a proper mental attitude backed by confidence, perseverance and courage. Despite all your shortcomings you will reach your destination. It is only through and by these traits that you will be able to weather life's stormy seas and bring your life ship safely to the port of fulfillment. And you will never hit a hole in one if you don't play! Here's a tip that may help…

Take your written life plan (you do have one, right?) and work it out to a definitive and successful conclusion in your mind. What does success in life really look like to you? One of my favorite authors, Mark Twain, wrote many years ago "let us endeavor to live so that when we come to die even the undertaker will be sorry!" That can be your story in a nutshell. Counseling that practice makes for perfection is simply declaring confidence plus perseverance equals victory. People who fail usually give up far too easily and far too quickly. You can't surmount your obstacles in life without exerting real and consistent effort. Nothing replaces persistence!

The word 'effort' really means the same as perseverance to me. Cowards are the only humans who actually quit in life's short race. In the handicapped world very few are cowards. I have counseled in my writings and public addresses that a smile is an asset no man can be afford to be without. It's true. A smile and a sense of humor has helped me overcome many trying barriers in life and it will do as much for you. Of course if you can't find your

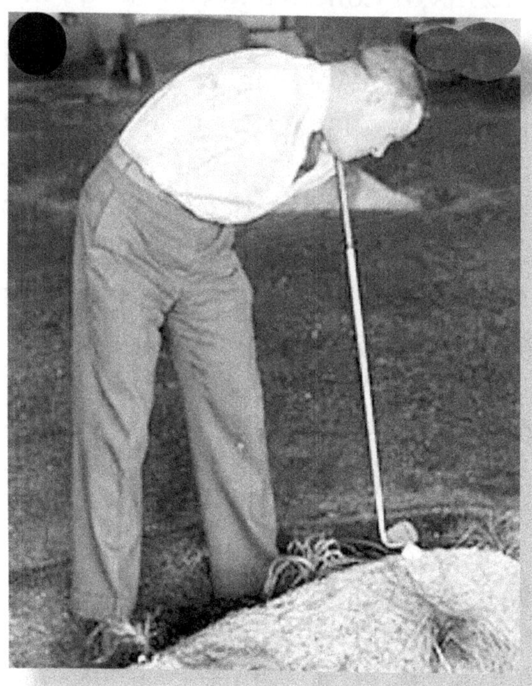

smile and you're going to sit idly by just because things are tough for you or because you can't get the things you desire immediately, than just a certain as I have no arms, life will quickly pass you by and suddenly without warning you will be merely a spectator in the defeated Gallery.

On the other hand if through confidence and effort you will say "I can" and say "I will" then life will indeed smile upon you with a full cloak of victory. Friends, as your sincere advisor I want to warn you that you can't afford to step out of line for a second. Sticking to a set course charted by yourself, with a proper mental attitude and a smile on your face with courage and faith in your heart, and with confidence and perseverance foremost in your mind, you will reach your destination and definition of success. Easier said than done I know, but do it we must.

Victory and success to many individuals are measured only in terms of dollars and cents. I do not subscribe fully to this belief because money won't buy personality, health, will power, courage, faith, hope or love. I know too many rich men who are miserable. Hard work and doing good and being productive and being a full man or woman, your efforts will purchase these things for you as they cannot be purchased with money. Money is not the all essential to make you happy. I know many, many miserable millionaires. Earning happiness is far more beneficial and should your goal be simply the gathering of money ultimately it will not profit you. Consider the words of Horus Green who once said "the darkest hour in any man's life is when he sits down to plan how to get money without earning it." I think he used to work in Government. To me the words 'swing' and 'perseverance' mean almost the very same thing. If you have a good Golf swing you simply follow through and if you have perseverance in life you do the same thing. In the battle of life you can't gain victory without them any more than a fighter, a Golfer or a baseball team could do so.

As a whole the handicapped fraternity have proven beyond question to a doubting world that they are blessed with a par level swing. This true fact is because the physically imperfect have been forced to deal with the fact that they have been knocked down more often and harder than a regular person. But it's their ability to get up, dust themselves off and always be smiling that allow them to always move forward. I appreciate fully that the physically challenged have a winning swing. However I offer the following poem to them and their physically perfect brethren for careful consideration. Friends, and I use the word in all sincerity, here's hoping you will find each line full of wisdom.

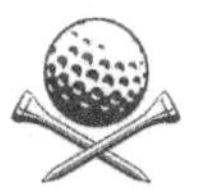

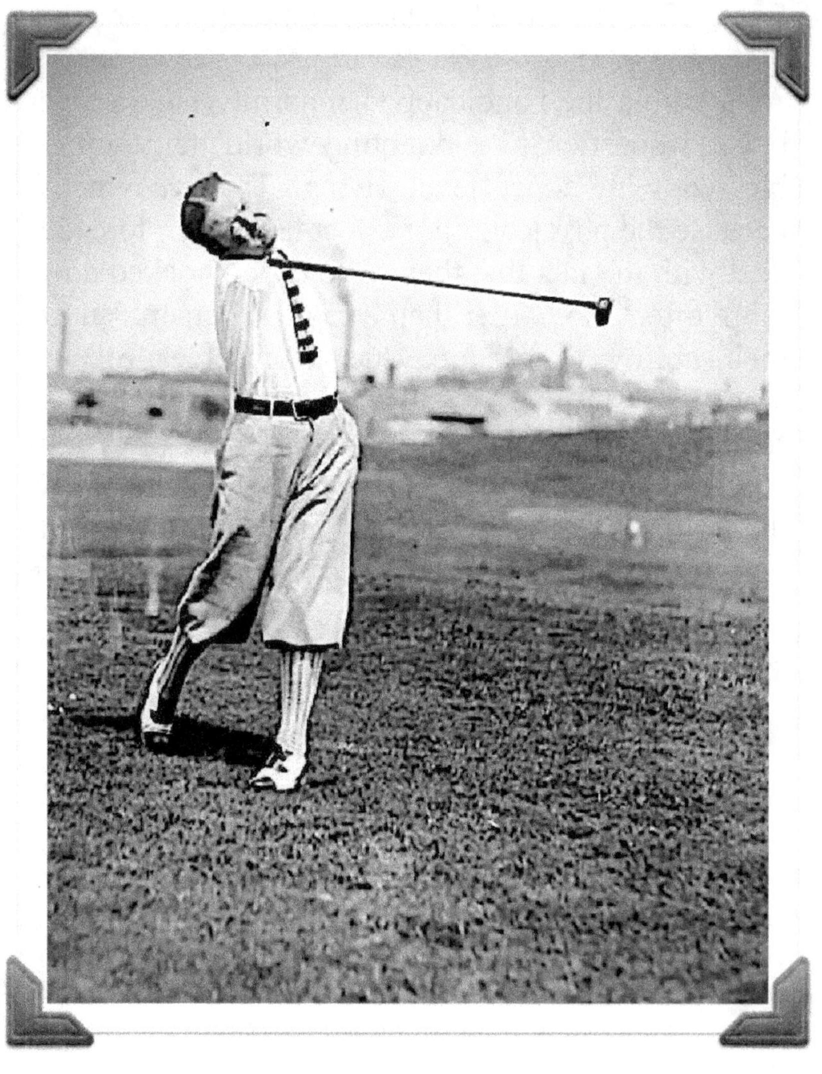

CHAPTER 9

The Swing of It
Nothing Ventured Nothing Gained

*"Golf can best be defined as
an endless series of tragedies
obscured by the occasional miracle."*
Arnold Palmer

A college education and its resulting degree was one of the things in life that I deeply longed for and cherished. I believed it was the salvation of my being able to earn a decent living. My dream was on the road to realization when my mother scraped together enough money to send me to Michigan State University. I wanted that college training to better equip me for life's battles. I pictured in my mind my diploma hanging on the wall with a big bold 'BS' after my name. Certainly those who'd seen my golf game over the years would think so!

I hoped against hope that it would be possible for me to earn a diploma. However my hopes were smashed when I had to leave school in 1915 not because of my grades, they were above standard, but only because my family could no longer afford the necessary dollars for me to continue. A sad state of affairs in the richest country in the world. With tear filled eyes and a very heavy heart I returned to our humble Homestead. Yes the one right across from the golf course. I felt badly about it naturally, and my mother apologized to me endlessly. I assured her that it was all right because I felt in my own heart that although we were still very poor I am still one of the luckiest men in America.

I console myself and have come to feel that it was all for the best and to this day I have no regrets because when that door closed other doors opened. Finding a paying job was my next task but what could an armless man do for a living? This was what I repeatedly asked myself. I had no arms but I'm proud of myself having good gray matter and a good sense of humor. My first job for actual weekly wages was with the Recreation Department of the City. Having been active in political and civic affairs I contacted my party and was put to work. I was told that my new job was one of the best in the Department.

Well imagine my surprise when I opened my Pay Envelope and found that the "best job" was compensating me at the rate of only $1.75 per day. I knew for a fact that another fellow, with the same job responsibilities, was getting three times as much. Although the work required of me did not require hands I suppose the "Head Man" figured that all an armless man was worth. Evidently they had not learned that it's one's mind and its proper use that makes for success, happiness and greatness. The $1.75 per day consideration got me to thinking, and for want of a better job I continued at work while searching.

Day by day I convinced myself that the 'head men', the guys in suits with new Chevy's in the parking lot, were wrong. In the future I would prove to a doubting world that the lack of arms would not deprive me of earning at least a decent living wage. I wanted to climb to the top rung of life's success ladder. I vowed that whenever the opportunity presented itself I would use my energy and my talents to convince employers that the physically handicapped are fully capable of doing an honest day's work for an honest day's pay. I hope you, dear reader, will help with that effort. With the physically handicapped and the thousands of war vets to come our country needs to open its heart and mind to this sector of our citizenry and use it for the productive resource it is.

Every citizen, every employer every new business owner should agree that there should be fair wage and opportunity for all in spite of any real or perceived handicap. We should make this the law of the land and we will. No greater stretch of the imagination is required to be convinced that the Depression has had a mostly devastating effect on employment including the physically handicapped. Depressions mean many things but unemployment is our chief concern and it is of course more acute in the placement of those physically handicapped individuals. That should be of concern for everyone.

And as we enter World War II it is natural that during the Depression and after a war, jobs become more scarce which makes it even more difficult. As I write this the Depression has been replaced with a modicum of prosperity and the "just around the corner" mindset has had its effect on everyone especially the physically imperfect. Even with the improving economy it has been nearly impossible to find gainful employment for the physically handicapped. No one, more than the businessman or the idle individual, need to be reminded that unemployed human beings are assets. Truly they are badly damaged citizens floundering about aimlessly in a lost market. Regrettably yet true, and through no fault of the individual, these folks can be and are rightly labeled unusable, and rejected. What a waste! In their own personal lives the unemployed have experienced these immeasurable hardships and the public now realizes the situation fully. We are filled with fear and we have too much sorrow over it. Being fully aware of these facts it's only fair and logical that you and I realize that the physically handicapped I have always been unemployed in good as well as bad times. I wonder if you've ever looked at this picture in just this light?

The Depression was nothing new for the physically handicapped as we have been in a perpetual one. Depressions mean many things. Unemployment is our chief concern and during this or any Depression unemployment is always more acute. Placement of those physically handicapped should be the concern of everyone. And it falls naturally that during any Depression jobs are more scarce. When everyone is affected equally it is hardship shared. If America enters the war there will plenty of work for everybody and those that are physically challenged still want a chance to serve our great nation.

Being aware of these unhealthy factors it seems to me a lasting asset should and could evolve. At least it gives me courage to suggest that from this day forward the handicapped of our United States should be taken fully into the circle of employment and made a tangible asset and segment of our society.

This is indeed asking very little. As a matter of record the clouds of despair and depression are slowly but surely lifting from our nation's bent shoulders. We now have another challenge before us which is to make the world safe for democracy, and handicapped individuals want and need to be part of this fight. Our unlimited patience and the spirit to carry crowns of hardship and never take no for an answer make us a natural asset. When the cause is

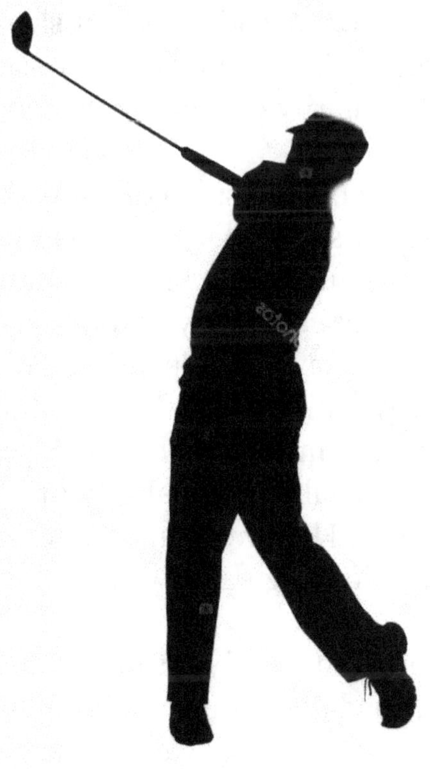

right and just the courage and perseverance to push forward has clearly been demonstrated by handicapped people. The handicapped should be made part of the team. I realize only too well that the greatest additional Handicap the physically imperfect face is the attitude of our fellow citizens.

There are those among us who think of the handicapped in terms of brooms, chairs, pencils and sideshows. Let them meet me on the Golf Course! Industry has a duty towards the handicapped from a social, economic and moral viewpoint. I recognize that there are others on the other side of the aisle who don't believe that. But we will reach a healthier national condition to have industry, of their own volition, absorb their fair share of the handicapped into their respective businesses and that'll be done voluntarily or by force of congressional action.

If the businessman of today can learn this lesson then I see the Depression as having been a blessing in disguise for mankind. During my service with the airplane company I won several Liberty Bonds for efficiency in competition with a supposedly superior armed individual. As I recall the airplane employment episode it amuses me but it is sad that it is typical of the majority of employment managers today. Here was a man offering me sympathy and charity when all I wanted was to work.

Unquestionably his heart was in the right place. But he had not learned what studies have shown, that physically handicapped people make capable, efficient and loyal employees. He did not know that 99.9% of the handicapped community do not court sympathy or charity. I have never courted either. Equal opportunities always, but sympathy? Never.

Generally speaking folks are too prone to showering sympathy upon individuals who through circumstances have lost their sight, become deaf or even lost both arms as I have. Besides, sympathy simply makes the giver feel better not the receiver. And let's not confuse sympathy with empathy. I speak from bitter personal experience when I say it tends to make the receiver weaker. I simply mean it tends to overdevelop the individual's sense of self-consciousness and lack of confidence. More often, it increases to the point of personal paralysis. It further instills in the individual the thought and feeling of helplessness and/or that somehow the physically handicapped can't measure up.

When you see a physically handicapped person, or any person with troubles that seem unbearable, don't shower sympathy upon them. Give them a word of encouragement and some empathetic understanding, a word of constructive criticism, but never sympathy. In Golf one must never offer criticism on the course, however sympathy often occurs.

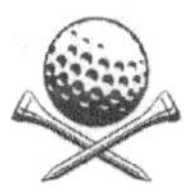

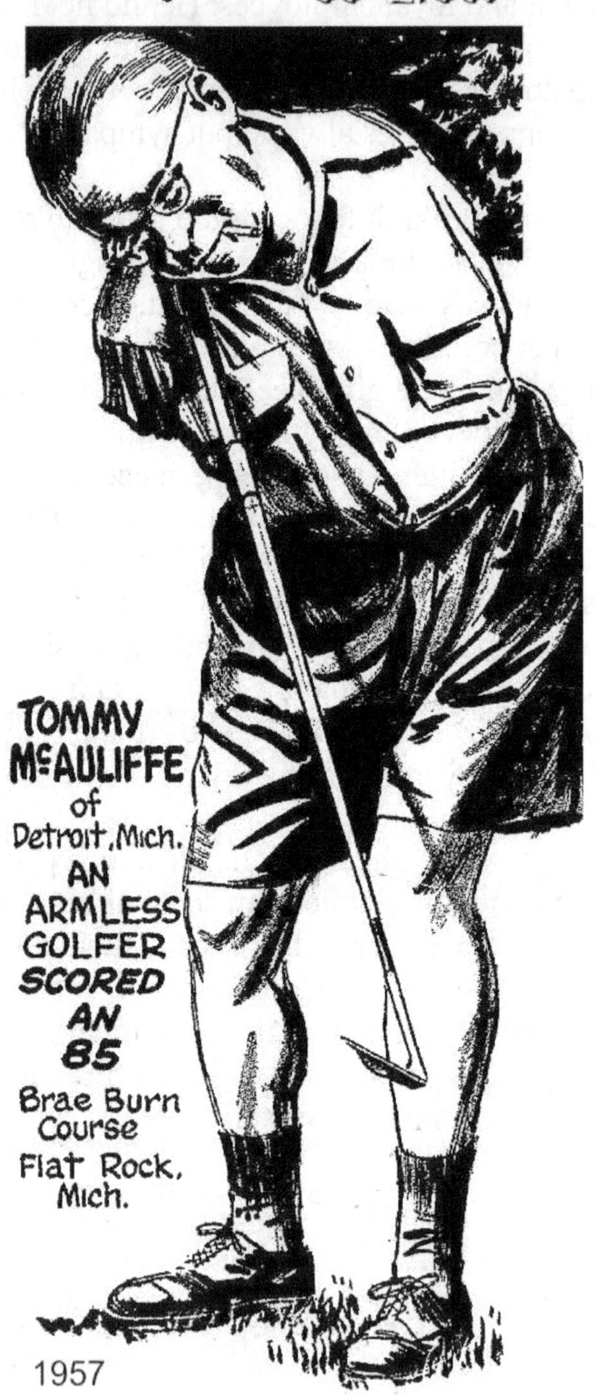
TOMMY
McAULIFFE
of
Detroit, Mich.
AN
ARMLESS
GOLFER
SCORED
AN
85
Brae Burn
Course
Flat Rock,
Mich.
1957

CHAPTER 10

Call a Mulligan
Sometimes Life is a 'Do Over'

"There's no movement in the golf swing so difficult that it can't be made even more difficult by diligent practice."
Tom Mulligan

"Always keep in mind that if God didn't want a man to have Mulligans, golf balls wouldn't come three to a package!"
Dan Jenkins

Perhaps big business labors under the false notion that an armless man is helpless. This attitude did not change my mental attitude nor was I embittered towards these merchants. It seems they knew "Tommy" too well. They looked down on me as a native son but they failed to grasp the full picture: I had grown to manhood and had produced in more ways than one, for them as well as my family and myself. You can't keep a good man down, as they say. Although no regrets lurk in my makeup, I should've worked as diligently as faithfully for myself as I did for them.

It seems as in many similar instances and circumstances, a native son must seek fame in other pastures before the Home folks realize the error of their ways. Being idle was no joke. I needed an income because things were desperate. My wife Marguerite took the fall with a full smile. She wanted to go look for a job but I would not encourage it. It was her faith in me, her daily words of encouragement, which kept me going from office to office and factory to factory. Something had to be done and done quick. And through it all as a soothing source of comfort and clarity was the timeless game of Golf.

So necessity was the factor which inaugurated my active show business golf career. Self-preservation and a decent living for my four children and their lovable mother was the necessity that instituted the invention. Forced to close the 'McAuliffe Coal and Ice company' and unable to induce anyone to give me a job, I was faced with a pair of alternatives… One, I could except charity and stay at home or two, I could take my golf clubs into Vaudeville and Show Business and be away from my home, and loved ones. It was no easy decision to make. I did not care for charity and I did not relish leaving the family. I discarded the charity idea immediately and decided to try the crazy business of show. Golf was one of the fastest growing sports in America at the time but Golf clubs in Vaudeville? On a stage!?

This was not my idea. My little brother Walter deserves that credit or blame. He had been doing amateur parts in theater and a short 'show' at gatherings around New York City. The skit was of such a nature that it could easily be modified to fit a

Golf act. He lost no time in doing this. So there we were with an idea, one old golf club and no modern stage experience. One golf club! What could go wrong? I did a little practice, chipping 13 balls into a bushel basket in the family parlor over and over. Practice was necessary because it had been years since I had actually swung a club consistently. I was too busy earning a living. After a little practice the old Mac returned. Naturally I was happy. Happy because I had found my swing again and happy that I could possibly make a living again, but still heavy at heart over leaving my family home alone.

All of this happened between Christmas of 1927 and January 1928, which just goes to show how quickly things can fall into place if you let them. By '29 guys in New York were jumping out of 11th floor windows, so I considered myself very lucky. We expect and demand from life more than we get. This expectancy proves that we are not acquainted with the true way to a joyous, happy and useful life. There is plenty of work for you and everyone else to do. It's a case of looking personally into one's inner self to ascertain if our machinery is running smoothly. Life for most individuals is a hunting program. First one thing is desired, then another, then something different again. This goes on year after year for even a lifetime.

Of course right minded human beings should strive for advancement, not just the appearance of progress. The man with or without a physical imperfection, should map out a definite life plan and stick to it. Stick to it every day, trying to improve over the previous day's living. And planning, whether it's a act for the Stage or 18 holes, is critical. Folks will tell you, for example, that when I play Golf I'm always thinking and planning two or three strokes ahead. You should too. But your life should not be one of continual hunting for this that or the other thing… fearful less you miss something or miss out on something. Beginning Golfers do that a lot. Instead of concentrating on finding their own authentic swing they try to copy a swing that is not theirs. They busily go from this grip to that swing and then something else and then back again and franticly think they are going to miss some secret approach or technique.

The individual who thinks he can't afford to miss things has not the faintest notion of how to live properly. In a handicapped life there are some things which must be foregone. In Golf you can't hit every shot well. In other words, the chap with the physical imperfection must forget his loss and begin at once to cultivate and use those factors he still has.

If you want to live fully, do not expect or demand from others anything, simply because you might have something to give in return. Would it not be better for you to view your brothers as they view you? If more of this were practiced our world, your life would be the richer because then, and only then, will it be possible for men to truly give something worthwhile to each other. This philosophy should be

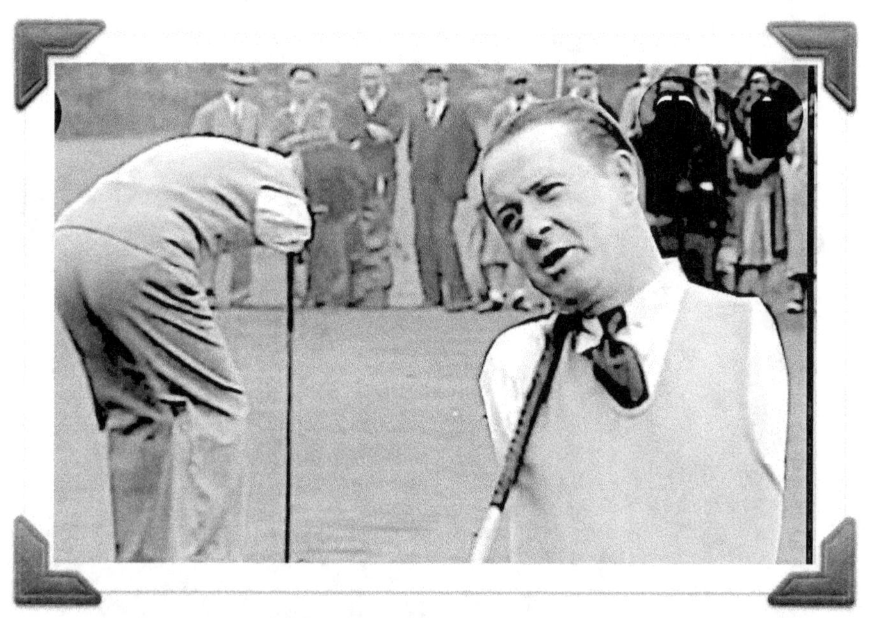

the daily watchword of every man and woman. 'What can I give my fellow man today?' If your life or your Golf match is not going the way you planned or wished it would, simply call a Mulligan! Start fresh and do a do over. After all you deserve it. But for some reason those on the road to rehabilitation and on the Golf course find it hard to forgive both ourselves and others.

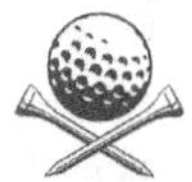

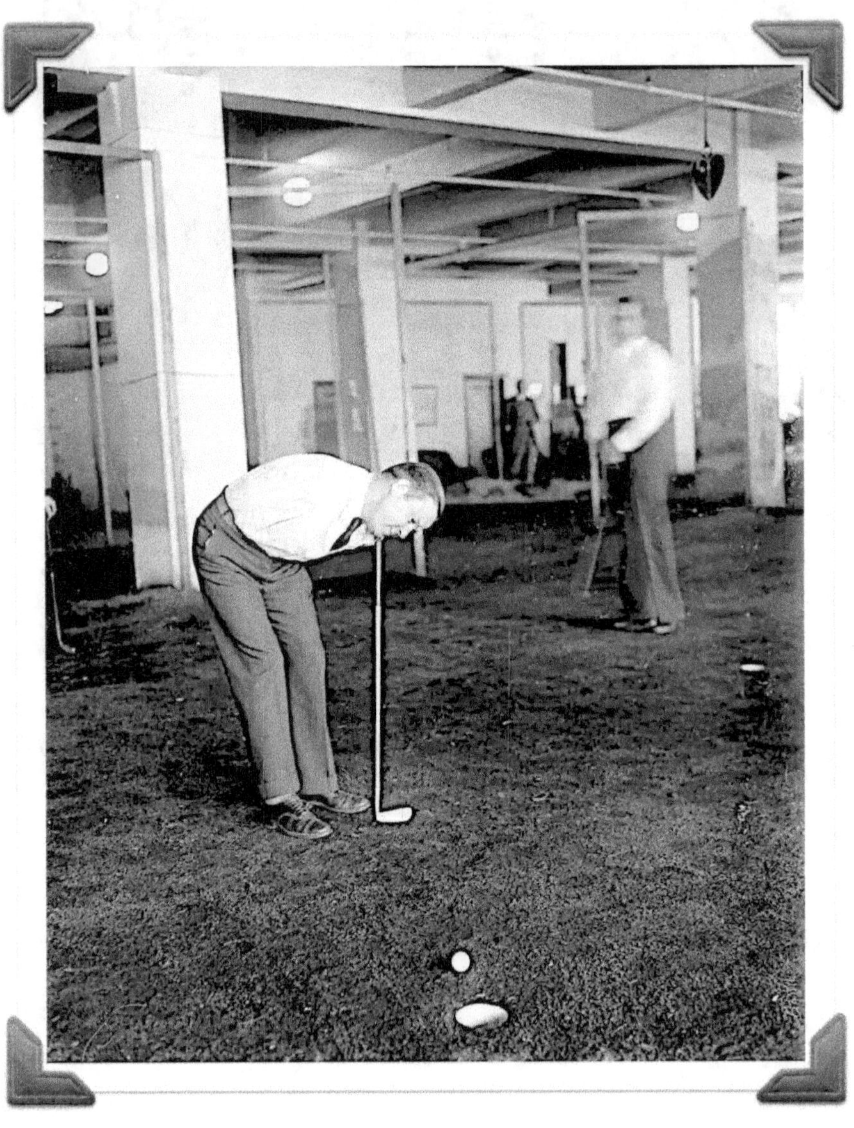

CHAPTER 11

Double Bogey
Every Failure Brings You Closer

"A smile will gain you ten more years of life."
Chinese Proverb

"No matter how bad you are playing, it is always possible to play worse."
Olympic Golfer Bobby Jones

The McAuliffe family was very happy with a new home in the Motor City. My friend, Golf legend Walter Hagen who lived in northern Michigan, had encouraged us to move due to all the opportunities there with the auto industry. We were getting a big kick out of our new car and we were truly enjoying life again after our first setback. All this enjoyment, all this happiness came as a result of my first Vaudeville tour which was a roaring success. It proved lucrative and enabled me to keep up the payments on our beautiful home.

I felt good that hard work and a few breaks could lead to the American dream… the fact I had no arms was not a factor. It was fun paying for our pleasure and gradually getting out of debt. We eagerly looked forward to the day when we could hold a family reunion around a huge bonfire in the backyard and burn the old mortgage. We were making progress because the mortgage on the home has been reduced from $15,000 to $8000 in just three years. It's important to set goals and make progress towards them every day and keep track of everything. I could tell you, for example, down to the penny how much per day I need to put aside to meet my monthly mortgage payment. Just like I can tell which way the ball will roll by the cut of the grass. Matters went along rosily until the fall of 1930, a result of the '29 crash no doubt. Then like a thief in the black of night the bottom fell out of show business. Folks simply could not afford a show at the local theater anymore and this new thing called Movies was changing the way people are entertained.

My agents in Chicago and New York City could not secure further bookings for me. Days, weeks and months went by and I took it all in stride, always keeping a smile on my face. Almost daily letters from my agent told me they were trying, and they would have something for me in a day or two. My other daily mail consisted of bills, bills and more bills from merchants who had been very kind in extending me credit. I had no money. Again, I was out of work. We had put every cent into over living and into the house but sadly and shortsightedly I had kept nothing significant for reserves.

I consider myself fairly smart but that was a huge mistake. Always pay yourself first was the lesson. My mental status was not the best, due to the bills and the high pressure collectors. calling and coming by the house. Having a strong mindset is vital in one's rehabilitation as well as the game of Golf as we've discussed. Then came a notice from the bank that they must have the money, actually only six months of interest, or they would foreclose on the home. At least they didn't want an arm and a leg! My back was to the wall in every respect. I tried to get someone to take my mortgage to give me a breathing spell but all I received was a negative reply. It was now the middle of 1931. I was given until September 1st to save my home. To whom do I turn? I knew not save for the one above…

I'm not ashamed to admit that on this and several other occasions my family would not have had food on the table if not for the extreme kindness of friends and relatives. To make matters worse the firm from whom I had purchased my household furniture was on my neck daily for money and threatened to back the truck up for the goods.

All in all it was not a happy outlook which confronted us. It would've been easy to just give up, throw in the towel and call it a day. But showbiz folks and Golfer are troopers. I lived an hourly prayer that somehow agents would come through with bookings or some other way to gain income. Some came but not enough and the thought of losing our home and its furnishings was also eating my darling wife's heart out. We were in trouble and I was frantic because I was truly helpless to do anything to prevent the promised foreclosures. And the feeling of helplessness, real or imagined can be one of the most disabling things that a person can face. But we did. On the 13th day of a solemn Catholic novena my wife and I were making, God suddenly answered our prayers. It was August 29, two days before deadline. It's funny how deadlines help focus the mind isn't it? I received a wire from Los Angeles offering me a full Vaudeville Tour with the famous Frenchon & Marco comedy and singing group. I was overcome with joy. And so were all my creditors! Now I could save our home and have something to bank on…At least for now.

Losing no time in contacting the bank, I was politely told, as only bankers know how to do, that unless I paid an additional $500 by tomorrow, they would have to put us out in the street. As a long-time customer. I argued and pleaded, mostly the latter, and told them I had secured work. I showed them the wire and my telegraphed acceptance, all to no avail. They might just as well have demanded the moon. I could've secured that just as easily as the demanded $500. However, they allowed us to stay in the house for a month, and October found us house renters again. Our savings had gone to the bankers. I relay all this simply to show you that everyone has hard shots in life. Everyone is hit with bills or illness or a terrible stroke, but it's how we respond to those things that makes the difference between a winner and a loser, a fulfilled person vs. someone wanting.

So onward I went into the glittering and cutthroat world of Show Business. My contract with the show production company had been signed. I was not scheduled to go to work until February but was guaranteed 32 weeks of work. The contract was shown to the head of the furniture house with the assurance that regular payments would begin immediately after I began work. It's true I was several months behind in the monthly payment of only $75, but I told my creditor that I owed very little compared to the original amount, so they should quote me some consideration. With hearts of stone they demanded $400 immediately or the merchandise. They suggested I go out and borrow it. One does not need to borrow money from a friend nor anyone else, I came to learn.

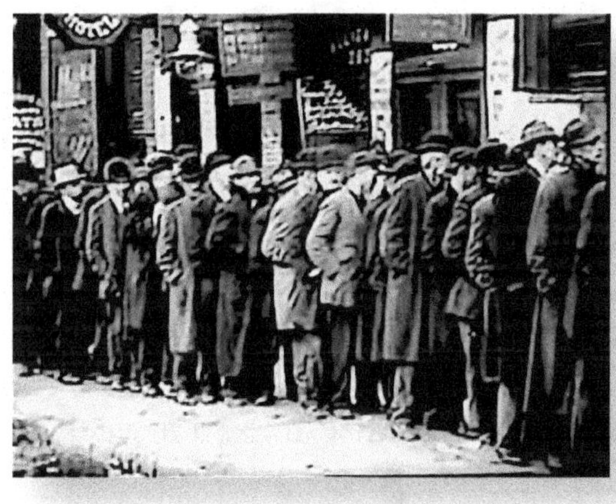

These especially trying times are nothing to what our nation went through during the Depression. There's no use crying over spilled milk they say, and that's especially true for financial matters. The savings of a lifetime were gone quickly, surely and undeniably. But it was part of life and I had faced tougher challenges. Just another sock on the chin. With my wife and family settled into a six room furnished flat I set out for the West Coast to fulfill my show business contract. I left New York on January 13, 1932 by train. Because of my financial circumstances and the state of the economy I accepted the tour at half my regular show fee. The tour required 42 exhausting weeks of travel to play the contracted 32 shows. I arrived home to my family just before Christmas in 1932 with exactly $100 profit from tour. For all the glamour, the newspaper and magazine articles, the Radio and theater appearances... and the time away from my precious family... Don't ever tell me that show business is easy. My homestay was not to be for long because my agents promised to have additional work for me within a couple of weeks. I was very pleased for I wanted to be with my family for the Christmas holidays and I wanted to play some Golf.

As January 1933 passed into history, I was still idle. The family money drawer was quickly dwindling. After paying the February rent there remained exactly 11 cents. With grateful thanks to my mother, we did not go hungry. On February 13 the senior district Director of Rehabilitation in the state of Michigan called at my house to tell me he had located a job for me with the County. I went to work that day at $16 a week. I got a raise to $20 a week that August and was named Assistant Executive Director in charge of the investigation department. Things were looking up.

The increased earnings made it possible to purchase much-needed clothing for my wife and kids. When the Federal Civil Works Administration (CWA) came into existence, I received more money per week, and during the life of our local CWA I handled nearly $2 million of federal funding. When an audit was performed, the next year they found that I was $.10 in the black. I was with CWA until 1935 when the Republican party gained control of the program and its board.

Shortly thereafter, I was removed for the insane reason that "I did not fit into the new executive director's vision of things". So I was idle again. Just another sock on the extended chin, and a good reason to always vote. Hard knocks form a vital part of life and Golf. They make us better and stronger. Show me somebody who has had it easy in life and usually I'll show you somebody with no character. At least hard knocks have been of value to me. I venture to say that had I not lost my arms I might not be as fulfilled as I am.

There comes a time in every life when you simply get downhearted, discouraged and blue. No one is perfect and troubles come along when they are least expected. That's why they call it a rainy day. But if handled properly, they can prove a blessing in disguise. When they come we're uncomfortable and often feel a bitter rebellion—why me? Some even have the thought of quitting life. Then that great and sure healer of all body and mental ills known to us as time, goes by and we are lifted up with the thought that things are fine with self and the world. Time can be your secret weapon. It heals all and provides a space to accomplish one's goals. If you have enough time, you can become accomplished at almost anything. The problem is most people never start or they don't practice enough to finish.

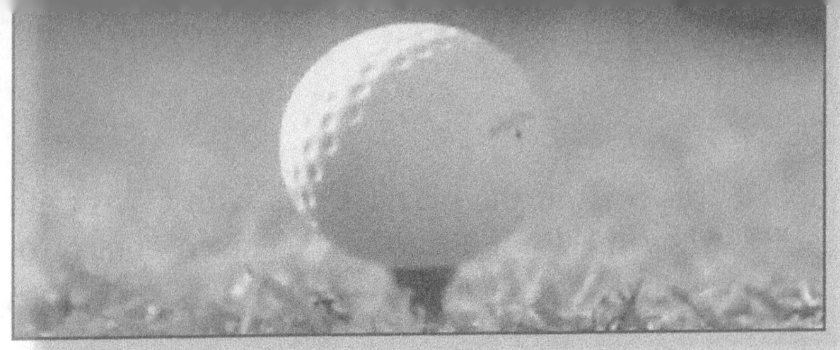

Cue the whiny voice… "Oh I'll never become any good". "Oh there's so many people who are better at it than I am" "I'll never win". If you start with that attitude, you're probably right. One is stronger because of the hard knocks, jolts and the bumps we receive traveling through life. Go back and re-read that sentence three times. When they occur, they seem unbearable at the time but we soon learn that they can be beaten by fighting on. When you emerge on the other side you're a bigger man or woman for having carried on. Simple. Or as I like to say; it's simple but not easy.

The bogeys meted out to us in life teach us the necessary attributes for success. They are patience and perseverance. I might throw in a third one and that is repetition. Successive refinement towards perfection has been my formula for success. We can't learn these lessons in any other way, it's the hard knocks that give us the experience of a most practical nature. True life experiences can't be garnered from this or any book. We must live them. The worthwhile things in life must be fought for and hard knocks are a necessary part of the process. Losing one's home, furniture and job was indeed a triple dose of hard knocks, a triple bogey of sorts, and of course it hurt. But when it occurred, I reverted to hope, that hope which told me that tomorrow would bring better things for me and mine. When most folks talk about hitting their knees and talking to the big man upstairs, invariably they ask for material things. Maybe I was a little different in that I always prayed for Faith. Hope springs eternal in the human heart, they say, for without hope, life would be indeed a drab affair. In fact there would be little incentive for one to carryon.

In proving the "no handicaps" philosophy, hope and faith played a vital role. They have been my guiding compass and this same faith has always lifted me up from the tough blows that came my way, be it losing both my arms to losing various jobs to losing my home. I would submit to you it's how I took these blows that made the difference. My hope has always convinced me that the best for me lies ahead. Faith is also like a vision and without that vision, my life would've been an empty one. Without a full dose of faith, I couldn't have proven "no handicaps".

To live life fully, every individual, regardless of race, creed, physical makeup or previous condition, must have a full measure of enduring hope and faith. Being out of employment only increased my supply of hope, and with that hope, I had faith in myself to go out and do the proper things that would lead me to success. I would have never reached the green if I didn't tee off and frankly there are many in this life who are simply afraid of failure so they never put the ball on the tee. You have a choice in life my friend. You can sit in the corner and cry over your lot in life or you can take the cards that life has dealt

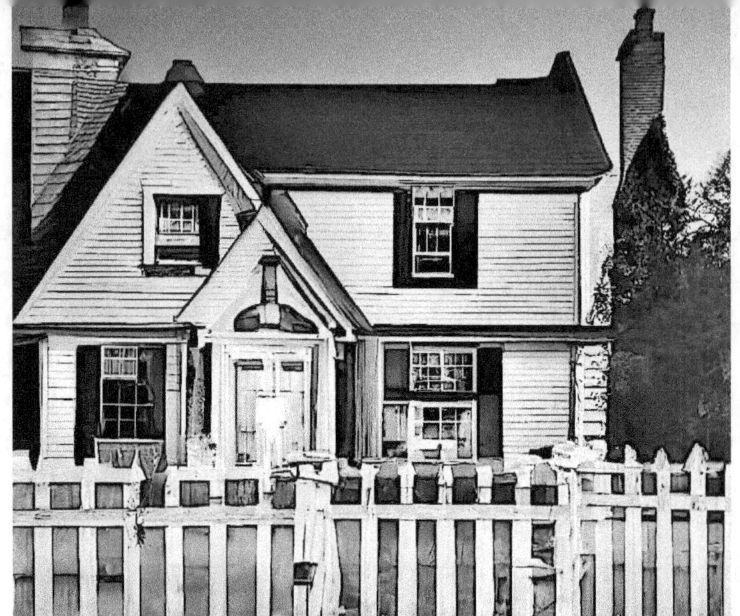

you and move forward. Anyway, the long and short of it is, try as I did, no job was forthcoming. However thanks to a friend, one of the finest sports writers and sports authorities in the United States, I was able to book some golf exhibitions around the country. The pay from these exhibitions was small but proved the means of keeping us from going hungry and naked.

With hope still firmly embedded in my optimistic heart I carried on and followed through. I knew my chance for real service to my fellow man would come someday. It was nearly the middle of July 1935, I was again idle but not discouraged, down but not out, because I was possessed with the feeling that the unexpected chance for real human service was about to come my way. I was about to take this double bogey of life turn it around and get back on the fairway towards the flag.

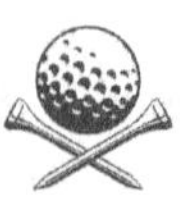

Chapter 12

Is that a Fact?
Fact vs. Opinion

"It ain't what you don't know that gets you into trouble. It's what ya know for sure that just ain't so."
Mark Twain

With 'No Handicaps' I have experienced and enjoyed many varied things in my interesting life. I have repeated many concepts throughout the manuscript because I have found that repetition brings memory and sometimes perfection. That is certainly true with the golf swing. Each swing is unique, almost like a fingerprint with no two exactly alike. As the new metal golf clubs came into being as World War II came to a close, the sport of Golf became more and more popular. We find that there are many ways to get on to the green, and that Golf swings are as diverse as the people that walk the planet.

Throughout this book you may have overlooked the consistent mention of the number 13. Despite thoughts to the contrary 13 has become my lucky number. In fact my show was initially called "13 Lucky Shots". Many things have happened to me relating to the number "13" over the years. I was born on Friday the 13th. The number of the streetcar that hit me was number 13. I was married on the 13th, mine was the 13th number called in the World War II draft, I was born in the 13th largest city in

America, I signed my first show business contract on the 13th, signed my Australian contract on the 13th, sailed for Sydney, Australia from San Francisco on the 13th, sailed for the United States and Los Angeles on the 13th. For some odd reason the number has been a part of my life. In my Vaudeville act there were 13 people on the stage. During my act I chipped 13 balls into a bushel basket and hit 13 balls into a targeted netted hoop.

They nominated me for State Senator on the 13th and the story appeared on the 13th page of the Newspaper. Superstitious? Not in the least. Superstition is simply fear in a person's makeup. I had courage, which is the antidote to fear. It's just a weird little coincidence. One of the most enjoyable facets of my pseudo-celebrity is being able to visit hospitals and rehabilitation centers for both veterans and children. One of the most enjoyable visits I have ever experienced was in May 1932 at the home for crippled children on Denson Avenue in Pittsburgh, Pennsylvania, USA.

Several days after that unforgettable visit I received more than 65 letters from patients there (the hospital specializes in children that have lost a limb). Columns of wonderful and lovely things have been written about me by members of America's greatest fraternity- the press. I fully appreciate all of them even though I humbly feel the compliments are not always fully deserved. Writing in the New York Times in October 1936 Columnist William Smith wrote about me: "Surely the career of world famous

Armless golfer Tommy McAuliffe should be an inspiration to every youth in our country. What boy ever entered upon a future life with such a disadvantage? Tommy overcame all his obstacles with a grin and a will to conquer. Good looking clean-cut and, to all other appearances, a normal young man. He makes an excellent public address. He has a personality that breeds confidence. That ever present smile wins the hearts of everyone. There is no man today who deserves the credit there is due Tommy McAuliffe. He alone won his fight.

The loss of his two arms at the age of nine itself was not the biggest problem it was the mental feeling of helplessness that is sure to permeate one's mind under such unfortunate conditions. Winning that battle takes perseverance. The compliment of every person in our country should go to him. He may

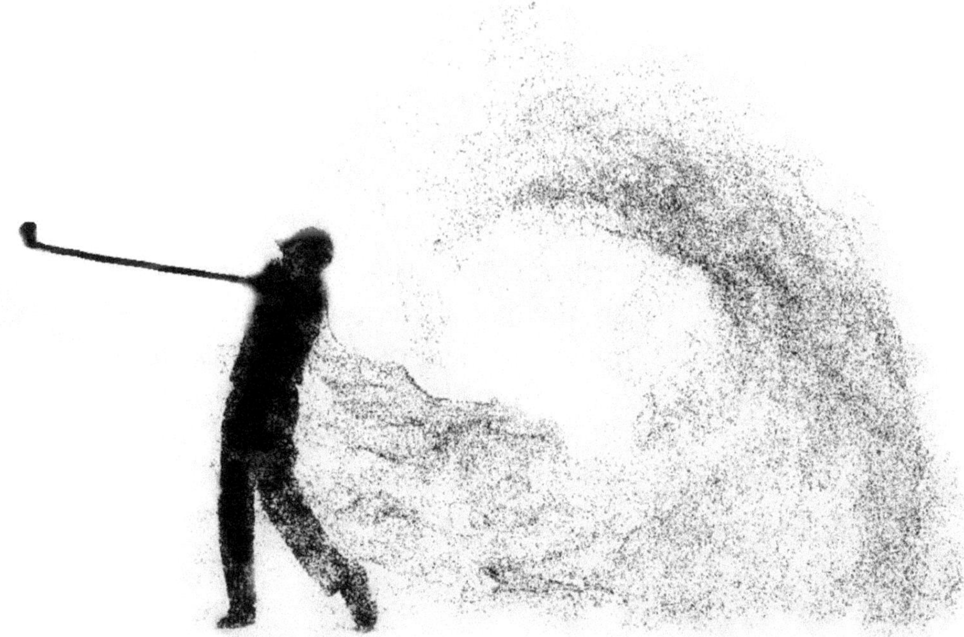

well be put on a pedestal as a model to American youth. He is a man's man." He certainly made me out to be something special. While I appreciate it, I don't agree with the 'good looking' statement because really my wife and kids merit that caption. However it was very nice of him to write it and I'll forever cherish his words.

Some years back when professional boxer Jimmy Slattery was tops in the light heavyweight division of boxing, he fought Maxi Rosenblum for the title. Now Maxi could only land a punch hard enough to break an egg. But Jimmy still lost the decision. Several weeks later I was at ringside for the Heavyweight Championship of the World fight. The day following, in the New York Times 'Before & After' column, was this comment on the previous evening: "One of the ringside incidents that made the bout easier to bear is worth repeating. Tommy McAuliffe, an armless Golfer just home from a Vaudeville tour around the country, was introduced. Tommy, dapper as Johnny Farrell, stepped into the ring, empty coat sleeves neatly pressed and tucked into the side pockets of his coat.

He took his introduction nicely and bowed to the rich ripple of applause that rose from inside the grandstand. When the hand clapping had partially subsided and Tommy was stepping from the ring, a shrill comment came from the shadow of the crowd and said, "put him in with Slattery!" I laughed myself silly. Jimmy Slattery was an excellent boxer. He lost because he lacked a real 'punch'… but not the kind with your fists, as he hit well. It's the kind of punch you need to gain life success. He needed the same "punch" to gain success in the roped arena. In short, he didn't think he could win—-so he didn't.

In proving "no handicaps" I have tried to have a punch in the fullest measure, in my lexicon it's "the swing." Golf is like boxing in some ways, but your opponent is yourself. Speaking to Rotary, Exchange, Kiwanis, K of C, Lions groups and various civic groups has always brought me pleasure. These organizations, in announcing my appearance, have invariably introduced me with flattering remarks, all of which I appreciate. I do hope that the hoopla does not diminish or disguise the method and philosophy of living life with 'no handicaps'. I have gone through life with empty coat sleeves, but I refuse to admit that I am handicapped and I don't really like the term 'Disabled'. I feel my record of achievement substantiates the statement that there really is no handicap but a mental one. From my career as a Journalist, as an Editor, a Golfer, an Actor and a Businessman, I believe I can do 99.5% of what a normal man can do. On stage when being introduced there is one thing I always insist upon… There must be no mention or even suggestion of sympathy. It's the one thing that I am sensitive about.

Sympathy has no place in my life nor in yours. "No handicaps" is without it. Sympathy, however well-meaning, is a deterrent factor in overcoming life's battles not only for the physically challenged but for the fully able as well. On my trip to the West Coast in 1932, I had the pleasure of addressing the large Kiwanis Club of Los Angeles, at which many of the foreign and United States Olympic games contestants were in attendance.

They asked me what one factor I felt made the difference between succeeding and failure, between winning and losing. It was the first time I've ever really been asked it in just that way and it took me aback a bit. I gave it some thought and the immediate answer I came back with is "spunk". You have to say to yourself, "I know they think I'm going to fail but I'm not going to lose and I have enough belief in myself to know what is a fact and what isn't a fact. Most people hear things and believe them, we are a trusting people. But many times, what folks believe are the facts are many times found not to be facts at all, they are merely conjecture.

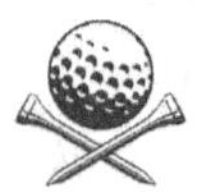

Chapter 13

The Creed of the Sans Arms Swing
Success = Repetition

"You're only here for a temporary visit. Don't hurry, don't worry. And be sure to smell the flowers along the way!"
Walter Hagen

"In Golf as in life, it's the follow-through that makes all the difference."
Tommy McAuliffe

Life, at best, is handicapped without a definite Creed. The full Definition of Creed is: "a set of fundamental beliefs and guiding principles." Never settle for mediocrity is one of my Creeds for example. I know fully that I am rather long in the tooth to have such a youthful Creed, but it has helped me, and I think others with similar situations. But this is what I believe and firmly advocate. It is not something that I share lightly and it is something that I have come to via direct experience, which I feel is the ultimate teacher. Doubt is around us everywhere. Always was and always will be. You and I are often bewildered. Often we find ourselves asking questions we've never asked before. Having doubts we never had before. And perhaps feeling a little bitterness. For what? To begin with, everywhere all around us there is an over abundance of suffering among the weak. Among the so-called strong we find stupidity, intolerance and indifference. Attitudes like this lead to a gloom and doom outlook. This is true not for just us individually but also for our nation. It's easy to sit on the sidelines and criticize others who are trying to improve their lives or our government.

One of the reasons I ran for public office was that I believe that if you want to complain, you have to take part. I feel that's true in Golf and that's true in life… If you want to win… you have to play! Doubt and depression and your disposition can dampen your physical and mental stamina. It can also really destroy one's helpfulness to oneself as well as others. Haven't you ever met someone who by all outward appearances should be down on their luck but somehow, through a friendly disposition, have made life not only just doable but actually fulfilling? It's a very sad state of affairs, but what is there for you and I to do?

Let's look at the picture through non-rose-colored glasses. If it were really depression, sickness, petulance, hatred or even war, we could deal with every one. History clearly proves those who are handicapped have faced all these things before and even more. But we had 'spunk' and we had a good swing and if we had guts, we fought and we eventually won. Of course we can face it again and again, but our problem is bigger than all these things combined, it is our outlook on life itself. I allude to the creeping cloud of doubt, which is about us everywhere, every day. It may prove our own undoing. It says, 'you can't', 'you won't', 'you don't'. What are we going to do about it?

My friends, there is a way, a very definite way forward. It has worked for me and if you will, but try, I believe it will work for you. I'm sure it will do at least something positive for you. And that is worth your full effort. Honestly, it's all very simple. But sometimes the simple things in life are hardest to accept and understand. Your initial internal reflection will disclose the fact that it's the simple things in life that count. That's what makes it worthwhile and more interesting. So then, my fellow Golfers in life, we must face the Fairway and when doing so have faith in ourselves.

First, take stock of yourself and instead of kidding yourself, be truthful. Don't deny the facts as they actually exist, don't blame the other fellow. If I had done these things, and I was tempted, I would be sitting on a front porch watching life go by. It's easy to go about shouting that this old world is going to hell in a hand-basket blaming all of your problems on society or Uncle Sam. Perhaps things for you are not as they should be or as you would like them to be. Well, what of it? Remember, there are others in the same boat. Others in boats that will find the bottom of Davy Jones' locker faster than yours, unless you and they do something about it.

Being paralyzed from analysis is something we should also guard against. It's easy to sit back and try and analyze a problem from various angles, but until you start to put forth effort in its solution, it is all for nothing. Without restraint, face the facts, and all of the facts, not just some. We must face all the facts large and small, real or imagined. Granted, things may look black or even hopeless for you, but it is only the light that makes the darkness disappear.

A coward is a product of the darkness, but faith in yourself is the antidote to doubt, gloom, despair and a half-hearted life. When you hit the Golf ball just right it's called hitting the 'sweet spot' and you can feel it in your bones. It is a true and pure feeling and connection with the ball. When you decide to live life with "no handicaps", life can indeed be sweet. Sure, it's sometimes a valley of tears, but it's the trying makes all the difference. When the valley of tears is full to the brim and you are at the point of disaster, take yourself by the hand and quietly go to your room.

When you are in your room or quiet place, talk to yourself not in softness or in terms of milky kindness, but with the iron hand of confession that you have been wrong in committing acts of meanness, selfishness, stupidity, vulgarity and cowardice. Only by owning up to our shortcomings and being honest about them can we correct them and move forward. If a man has a slice in his Golf swing and won't recognize it and try to work on it, he can still enjoy the game but he will never fully enjoy it like someone who is taking the time to master driving a straight shot down the fairway.

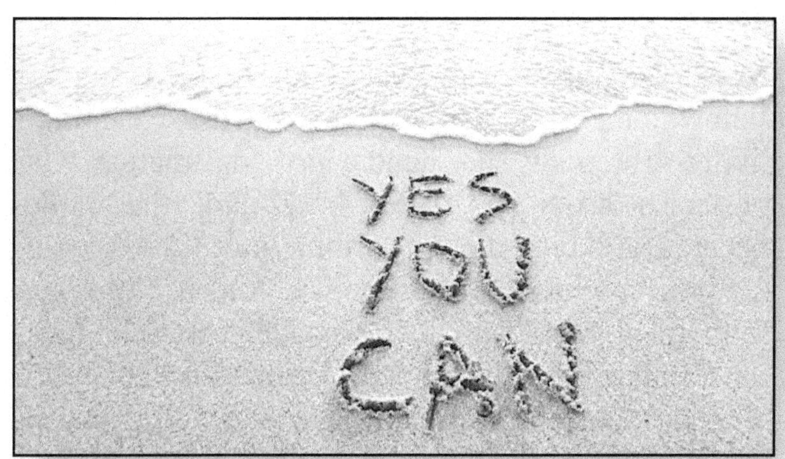

Recognizing our shortcomings, we begin to realize that makes us realize we are bigger and better than our past mistakes and that our earthly carcass holds finer acts which are yet to come. Let your fellow man look down upon you in scorn and let the entire world turn against you because if you have faith in yourself, you will be the winner in the end, regardless. Faith in yourself is consoling and satisfying. However, there is something or someone most of us know little or nothing about; it's God or Buddha or Mohammed or some other deity. Whatever works for you. To me, it's God and there are many paths to his house.

Many times when something miraculous happened in my life, things I couldn't explain, I knew that there must be some unseen hand guiding me along the way. We all have different beliefs of what God is, but I believe there is a God. I haven't seen him nor can I prove he exists, but I have faith in him since the day I looked up from those train tracks.

My dream, my vision, my faith in God and my fellow man is to allow all to see the wisdom in living life with "no handicaps," no matter what obstacles arise no matter how dark the clouds become, and regardless how long or crooked the dog leg hole might be. I still believe. And if I can have faith in myself, faith in God, then certainly I can have faith in my fellow man. I often think that God could've taken my life on the streetcar tracks that fateful day so long ago… But He didn't. So through my positive attitude, I have found that yes life can indeed be sweet. These principles are what have enabled me to prove to myself and to others that there are no handicaps in life except mental ones. The game of golf has also taught me life principles that are real, true and understandable. I predicate this outlook upon my deep belief and experience that there is no handicap in life except for mental one… Seems you've heard that before right? This is not only my belief, but is my creed and my sound philosophy. I hope it will help you in playing the great game of life and one of the most frustrating sports ever invented. The summation is that we get out of life all the good things in beauty and success we deserve based on our efforts.

When I lost both arms, it would have been simple to sit in the corner and cry about it to sit back and do nothing to help myself to say to myself "What's the use, my parents will take care of me and when they're gone it will be up to the state to do the same." But I've become happy in what I've been able to do in my humble way, and my course was a hard one at the same time. As I reflect in retrospect, I am convinced it was the easiest way. At least it proved a happy, productive, and a satisfying 18 holes.

Naturally, losing a couple of arms was a terrible blow. Gone were my dreams of ever becoming a big league baseball pitcher or pro golfer. Just because I was void of a proper mental attitude, I sometimes saw in myself the idea that everything worthwhile in life for me was gone. My situation at the time upon return from the hospital was like the story of Pat and Mike. These Irish buddies were constantly arguing about religion. Pat was a devout Christian, believed in heaven and hell, and Mike being a disbeliever, declared that neither place existed. This argument went on for years. Mike passed away and was laid out for the funeral in his best full evening-wear. Pat was very sad and he went the first night of the week to pay his last respects.

There was no one in the parlor except the corpse and after a few silent prayers Pat stood at the casket in silence, gazing at his friend Mike in full regalia. After a long silence, Pat said aloud, "well Mike, you didn't believe in heaven and hell so here you are… All dressed up and no place to go!" In the round of life I too was all dressed up with no place to go because I was lacking a proper mental attitude that mental attitude that would assist me to make molehills out of my problems instead of mountains. Unfortunately, this world of ours is replete with men like Mike. Through a proper mental attitude, I have made mole hills of all my problems. Like my golf swing, this has only been possible through cultivation and repetition. Believing one can makes all the difference and this alone has made 'no handicaps' a reality.

Ever since I was a lad I have desired someday holding office. In 1926 I tried to realize this ambition by seeking election as a state senator. Naturally I was defeated, but I was not disgraced and the issues we brought up here in the campaign were needed and substantial. Defeats were and are nothing new to me, and I learned that public service was not to be my calling. I'm interested in helping people take new courage, be renewed and then play the game of life. Through Golf I have both entertained people and learned lifelong lessons on how to both live a fulfilling life and be a better citizen. I'm happy in the thought that mine is the opportunity to give people food for thought in solving life's problem. This philosophy has helped me and I believe if it is followed and practiced by you, it will prove an asset to you.

The best golfer to play in the 1930s arguably was Henry Picard. During the decade, he won two majors, including the 1938 Masters Tournament and the 1939 PGA Championship. Picard would end the

1930s with an impressive total of 26 wins, and I think if you would have asked him, as I did, what his secret was, he would again say it was a strong mental attitude. On the tee and green, his concentration was legendary. This world is yours for a struggle. There are hundreds of thousands of humans more poorly equipped than you. If I could get up after being deprived of both arms, go successfully through school without asking special favors, learn to write with a paper, pen and typewriter, and do all the other things in life that make life worth living, then surely you can too. And learning to play near par Golf has also taught me life lessons of patience, perseverance and community.

I refused to be licked by not having a couple of arms so why should you not make a greater success of your life or your Golf game by having a full mental and physical inventory of your strengths and weaknesses. You'll find that the only handicap one has it's all in the mind. It's a simple but not easy concept to come to grips with. With a strong mental attitude, you need nothing more. Make courage and consistency yours to the fullest and you too will prove "no handicaps" not just in Golf but in your life as well. May you hit life's ball straight down the fairway of life and directly into the cup!

The End

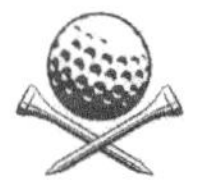

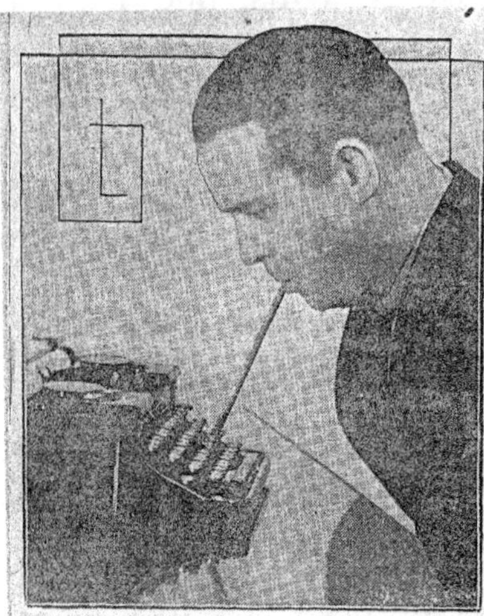

TOMMY M'AULIFFE

The picture shows Tommy McAuliffe, armless golfer, who will entertain at Tiedtke's food show this week. Tommy can operate a typewriter with a pencil held between his teeth.

* * * * * *

WHAT was surely the strangest golf match ever played was staged at Dorchester, Mass., recently, when Joe Sweeney, Boston's famous one-armed golfer, played a round with Tom McAuliffe, Buffalo's armless player. A large gallery followed the unique match and enthusiastically cheered the courage of the sportsmen who have surmounted unusual handicaps. McAuliffe won, 94 to 96, medal play.

* * * * * *

BOSTON EVENING AMERICAN WEDNESDAY, APRIL 20, 193

NO ARM VS. 1 ARM AT GOLF

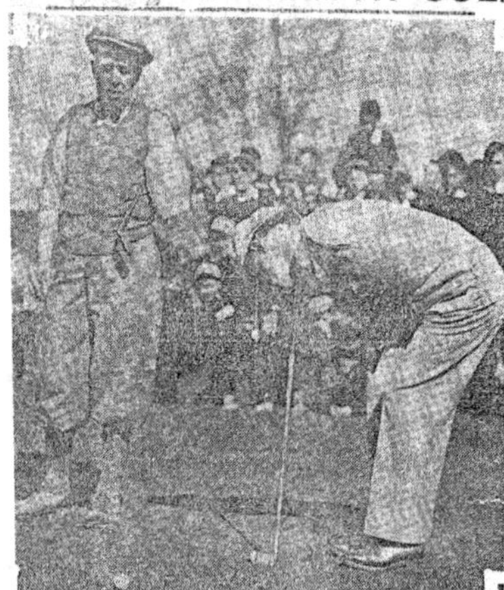

JOSEPH SWEENEY   TOM McAULIFFE

he strangest golf match ever beheld—a sight that would have gladdened the hearts of the Geneva disarmament conference—as witnessed on the Franklin Park links today when Joseph Sweeney, Boston's famous one-armed golfer, played Tom McAuliffe, the no-armed golf marvel, who is showing audiences the Metropolitan this week how he plays without h——

A food show was opened by Tiedtke's Monday. It will continue through Saturday.

Food manufacturers throughout the country, who are co-operating with Tiedtke's in conducting the show, have informed store officials that this show will be the largest to be held in any store between New York and Chicago.

Orange growers from California, several flour manufacturers, meat packers, cereal manufacturers, candy makers and others will have experts at the show for demonstration purposes, officials of the store said Monday. An oriental tea booth will be a feature. Souvenirs will be distributed.

Tommy McAuliffe, armless golfer on the Paramount bill this week, will be an added attraction for the food show. He will provide entertainment on Tiedtke's third floor Tuesday, Wednesday and Thursday. McAuliffe can make difficult shots at golf and can operate a typewriter with a pencil held between his teeth.

McAuliffe, an armless trick golf shot wizard furnishing many surprises. Earl Le Vere and Mildred Bryan in an eccentric comedy turn, win most of the laughs on the bill.

DETROIT FREE PRESS

Dancing, singing, acrobatics and skill in several directions feature the Fanchon and Marco idea "Stitch in Time," with Tommy McAuliffe, the armless golfer, to enthuse devotees of the game with his deftness. There is some delightful dancing by the Carla Torney girls and stepping of a different type by Benda Torao. Earl Lavere and Mildred Bryant in comedy patter; Harriet Mortimer, with songs, and the tumbling and juggling of the Five DeCardos, offer a diversity of talent. Popular torch songs are woven into an orchestra overture with Steve Weninger as soloist.

Loss of Arms No Handicap To McAuliffe

Armless Golf Wonder in Exhibition at Glenwood Links

IN golf handicaps are something to be overcome. In life, handicaps must be treated in much the same manner. At least Tommy McAuliffe, a young man who comes to the Glenwood golf club Thursday afternoon for an exhibition match, says so. Tommy overcame both physical and golf handicaps and is the only man in the world who plays golf, and good golf, without teh use of his arms. The reason for this is that both arms are off at the shoulders.

Tommy, not yet 30 years old, was but nine when a railroad train amputated both arms. In the years that followed he has successfully overcome all the obstacles and handicaps that have faced him both on the golf course and in everyday life.

A great game of golf is just the ordinary thing in Tommy's life. He drives 150 yards on an average. He was for 13 years a sports writer on a newspaper, and never missed an edition. Minus his arms, Tommy can write his name or any other words as legibly as anyone.

He says he has the advantage over most golfers inasmuch as he never has to worry over whether or not he is using his wrists properly, or wonder about which grip is the best, or fret about his follow through. McAuliffe has one grip and it always works. He breaks 90 on almost any course, no matter how difficult.

Tommy demonstrates far better than anyone can describe on paper. He is in reality a sort of phenomenon. His clubs are of regulation make and are equipped with no special apparatus to simplify holding. He uses no tricks, although his grip is necessarily a little different than that of the ordinary golfer. Tommy teaches a lesson in perserverance as well as expert and trick golfing.

Tickets for the match will be on sale at the local golf clubs as well as downtown agencies, to be announced later.

Trick Golfer

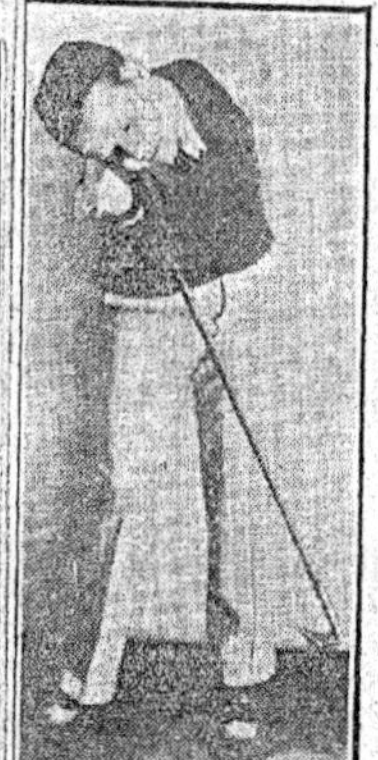

Tommy McAuliffe, who is seen in "Stitch in Time" at the Imperial Theatre. One of America's trick shot golfers, he plays without arms, striking the ball by holding his club between his neck and shoulders.

UNUSUAL MATCH AT HARTFORD GOLF

One of the strangest matches ever played on local fairways will get going Tuesday morning at the Hartford Golf club when Tommy McAuliffe, who lost both his arms in an accident, will nevertheless carry off his part in a foursome. Tommy swings clubs by his teeth—and, what is more, Tommy checks in some good scores.

The other three players, who will tee off at 10 a. m., are A. S. Beyriton, director of vocational education for the state board of education; the Hartford Golf club professional, Sid Covington, and Arthur B. McGinley, sports editor of The Hartford Times.

As part of his program this week in having Mr. McAuliffe demonstrate what handicapped men can do, E. P. Chester, the director of vocational rehabilitation for the state board of education, has arranged the golf match. In the interested "gallery" of state officials at the links Tuesday will be State Comptroller Frederick M. Salmon.

It is Mr. Chester's job to direct the work of rehabilitating handicapped men for a useful place in industry.

Tommy McAuliffe is appearing this week at the Capitol theater.

EXTRAS

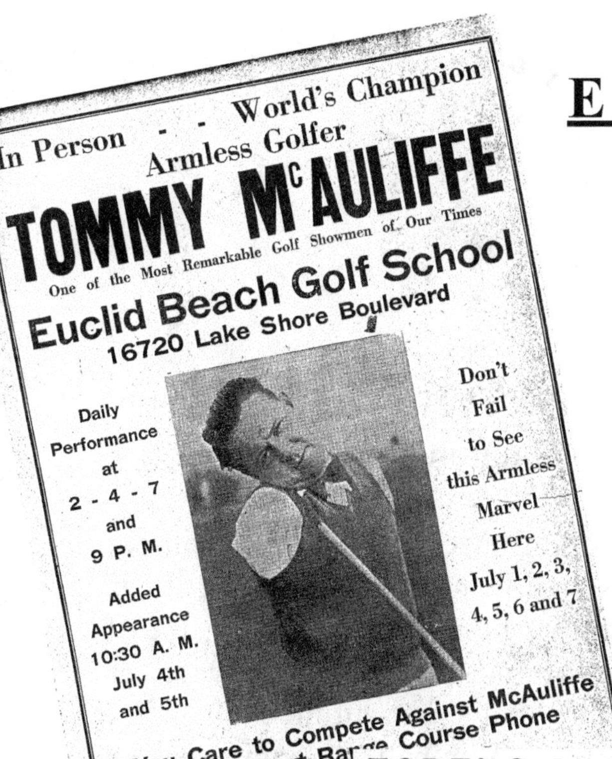

FORE! Golfers! FORE!

Clear The Fairway

for the one and only

TOMMY McAULIFFE

World's Champion Armless Golfer

NOW FEATURED AT THE

PARAMOUNT

T H E A T R E

In the Sparkling Stage Show

"STITCH IN TIME"

In His Own Inimitable Act

The General Public Is Invited To View

TOMMY McAULIFFE

TODAY
at
4:30 P. M.

on the main floor of our store
in a demonstration of
Golf Shots—unique
and orthodox!!

TODAY
at
4:30 P. M.

McAuliffe will inspire every Golfer to better play. See him DRIVE.....
watch him APPROACH....view him as he PUTTS....and then stare at
him as he goes through a repertoire of Trick Shots.......he's a wonder!

What McAuliffe Does With NO ARMS You Should Do With Two!

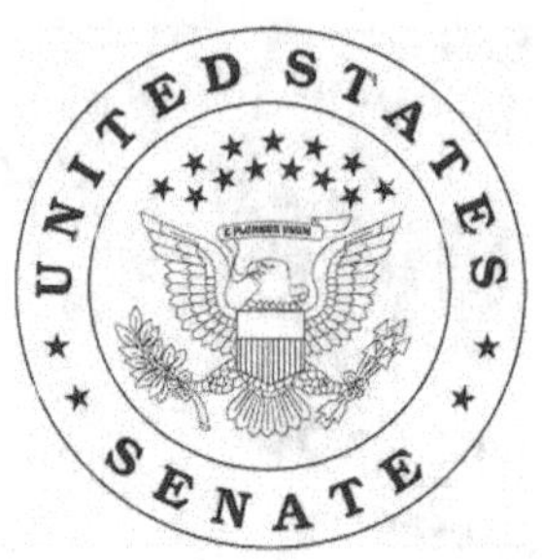

The United States Senate
Washington, DC

No one can hear Tommy McAuliffe's story without taking a new look at life most of us think life is pretty tough especially these days we find a lot of fault because things are not passed to us on a silver platter sometimes. If that's our attitude his story should put us to shame! With half our equipment he has twice the courage of any average man.

Is it pure selfishness or cowardice that makes so many of us consider that we have handicaps in the game of life? Be it physical or mentally? Why do we limit ourselves when a man without arms says "I have no handicaps!" This man overcame obstacles which would drive many a weak soul to suicide. Instead of morning and lamenting and wailing and worrying Tommy looked at life square in the face and brushed aside every natural instinct to loaf the rest of his days. His is the stuff of which legends are made.

What McAuliffe did should be an inspiration to every limited person in all the world. It should renew the enthusiasm of those who are striving for rehabilitation or just trying to live their best life. It's an outstanding example of what willpower can do.

World famous Blind, Deaf and Mute Helen Keller, who learned to communicate with the no assets and World Champion Armless Golfer Tommy McAuliffe are the King and Queen in the royal family of spunk! Their achievements are an inspiration.

If I had my way I should make Tommy McAuliffe a wandering evangelist traveling from institution to institution where cripple persons of the body or mind are found. But first we need to get him off the golf course! I would endow him so that he could spend the rest of his life seeking out and encouraging men and women who have suffered similar accidents. His example and courage will inspire others to go and do likewise.

My hat is off to World Champion Armless Golfer Tommy McAuliffe!

Senator Royal S. Copeland
United States Senate
D-NY
Chairman: Subcommittee on the Handicapped
1937

Read into the Congressional Record

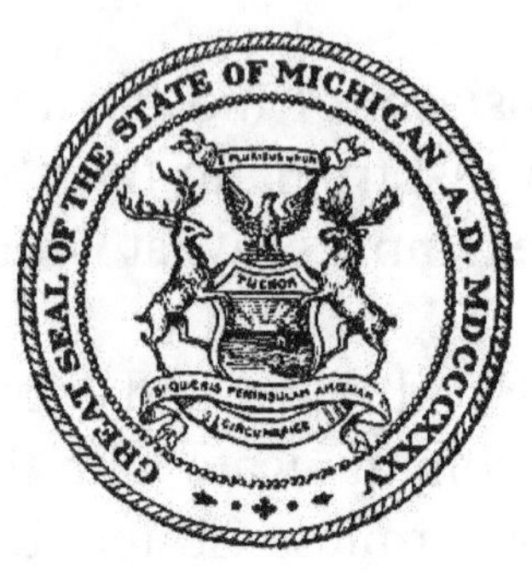

Let It Be Known…

That Tommy McAuliffe is 'the Rehab Man'! "I will succeed!" that's what you always say and do. Your 'No Handicaps' philosophy has and will help millions of disabled Veterans and the handicapped. You've always assumed you could succeed and you always say you will succeed not if I succeed, there are no 'maybes'. You've been met with many difficulties throughout life but you always meet them head on… you size up the challenge, plan your drive down the fairway and then follow through!

One of your fellow newsmen in Washington DC I think summed it up beautifully during his recent news column; "Tommy McAuliffe carries the empty coat sleeves tucked in the pockets of his coat… Not as a badge of defeat, but rather as an emblem of distinction." You have faith in yourself which is evident when you talk. You come from conviction with faith in yourself and the you are at par with any other person or group. You ask and accept no service that you can perform yourself. Your actions are an evidence of "no handicaps" because believing you have none you ask for no special favor; Not in business and not on the Golf Course. You always set high standards for yourself even with the presence of a physical disability great enough to render many a person utterly helpless. There's no excuse in your mind and there is no self-pity, self-consciousness or malingering in your make up.

The factors that have made your life a success and a reality are well expressed by writer Charles Dickens when he said "think hard, work constantly and make the best of things as they come along!

The self-realized methods you've learned to utilize have effected your success and have proven to be the backbone of any great rehabilitation plan. Professional or amateur these life tools may be used to advantage by both the physically disabled and the physically normal. Indeed I believe you've indeed created a new type of man, 'the rehab man', the rehabilitation man is a new man that despite any physical infirmity refuses to be 'less than' and won't take no for an answer. Those invisible arms you carry in your head you have learned to use well. Tommy McAuliffe, is an inspiration and a man to be respected in life, the Boardroom and Golf Course!

Gov. Frank Murphy
Michigan - D
1938-Governor's Proclamation

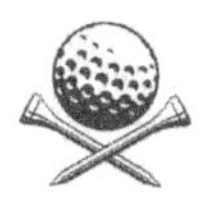

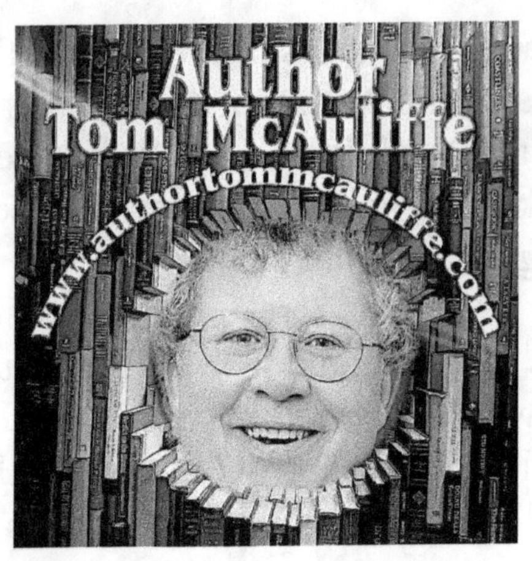

Please send questions to:
Bookinfo@nextstopparadise.com

Please Leave a Review!

Good or Bad they really help…

Member:

Alliance of Independent Authors

Emerald Coast Writers

Military Photojournalists Association

Florida Writers Association

Acknowledgments

Kissimmee Country Club, Florida

The USO

The United States Congress

Disabled American Veterans

Buffalo New York Sports Association

Ripley's Believe It or Not, Inc.

The McAuliffe Heritage Center, Ireland

DepositO Photos

Jim Bryant Photography

The McAuliffe & Tinney Families

The Associated Press / UPI

The PGA

Michigan State Medical School

Books by Author Tom McAuliffe

• Mr. Mulligan - The Life of Champion Armless
Golfer Tommy McAuliffe

• Nuts! - The Life & Times of Gen. Tony McAuliffe

• Throttle Up - Astronaut Teacher Christa McAuliffe

• Mad Dog! - Detroit Tiger Dick McAuliffe

• Charmed - From Motown to Combat & Back

• Almost - The Road to the Grande

• Thunder Road - Goodyear, God & Gatorade

• Buddy, Brian and Me - A Spooky Rock Story

• Frozen - A WWII and Mind over Matter Tale

• Soft Shell - Teddy the Talking Turtle

• Max & Me - Paws Across The Water

• Off the Rock - Escaping Alcatraz

• Deepwater Oil - Drillin on the Moon

• Books - eBooks - Audiobooks •
*On sale at Amazon, Kindle, Apple iBooks, Barnes &
Noble and your local independent book store!*

Also Available at:
WWW.AUTHORTOMMCAULIFFE.COM

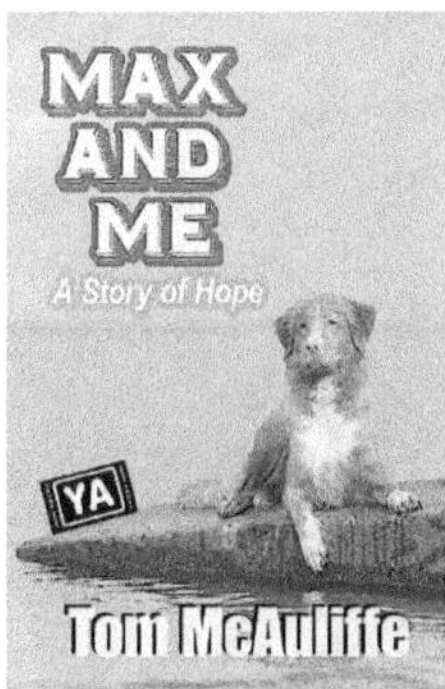
MAX AND ME
A Story of Hope
YA
Tom McAuliffe

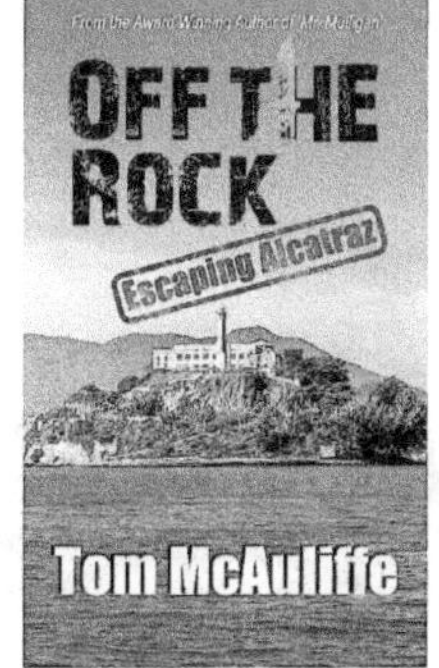
From the Award Winning Author of 'Mr. Mulligan'
OFF THE ROCK
Escaping Alcatraz
Tom McAuliffe

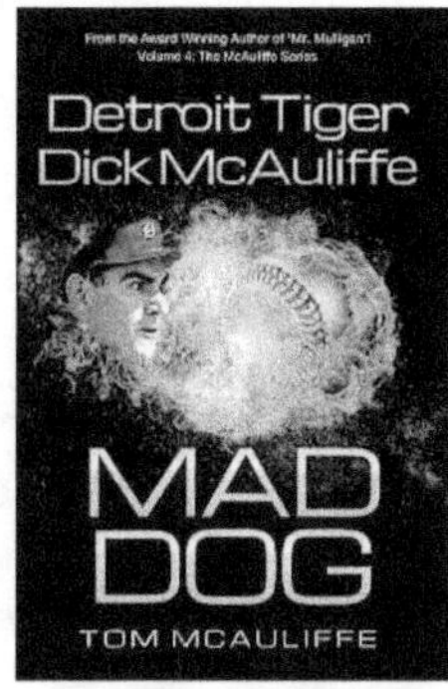
From the Award Winning Author of 'Mr. Mulligan'!
Volume 4: The McAuliffe Series
Detroit Tiger
Dick McAuliffe
MAD DOG
TOM MCAULIFFE

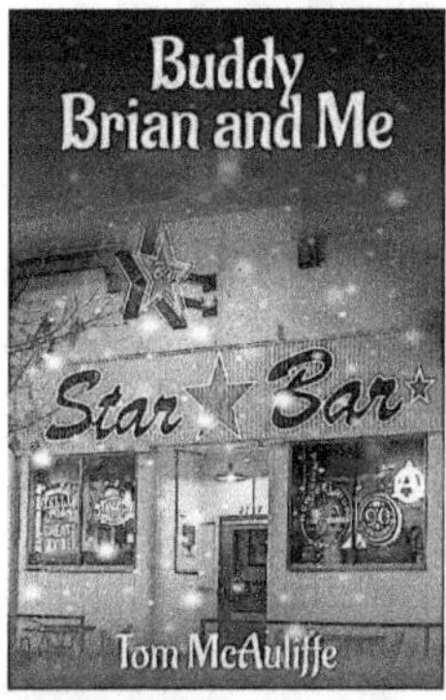
Buddy
Brian and Me
Star Bar
Tom McAuliffe

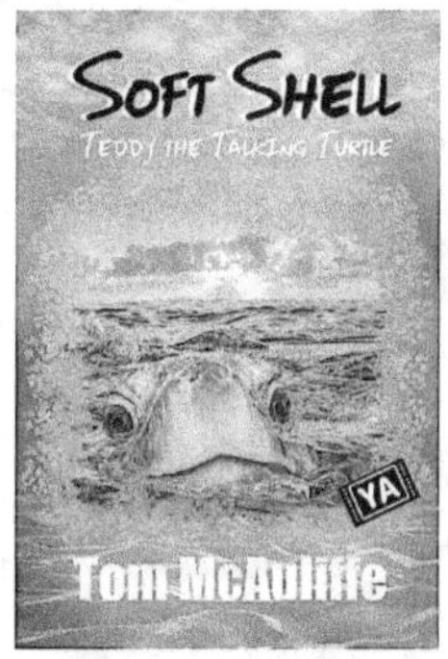
Soft Shell
TEDDY THE TALKING TURTLE
YA
Tom McAuliffe

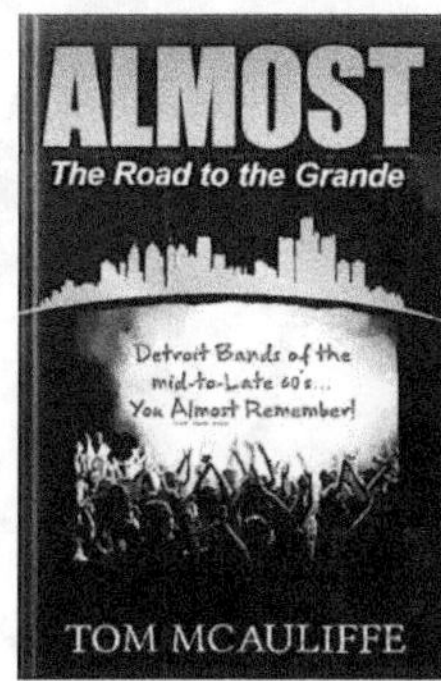
ALMOST
The Road to the Grande
Detroit Bands of the
mid-to-Late 60's...
You Almost Remember!
TOM MCAULIFFE

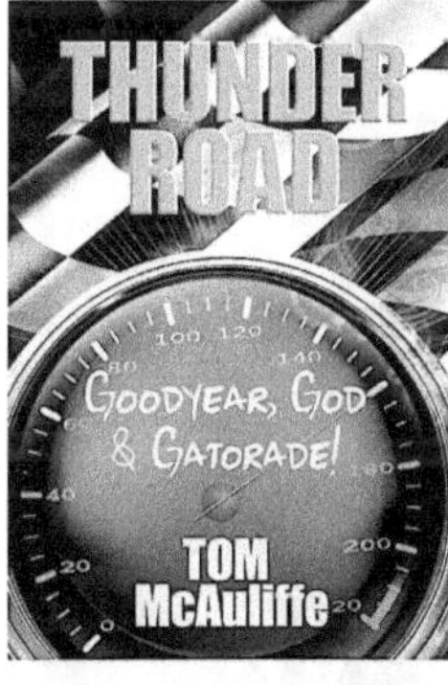
THUNDER
ROAD
GOODYEAR, GOD
& GATORADE!
TOM
McAuliffe

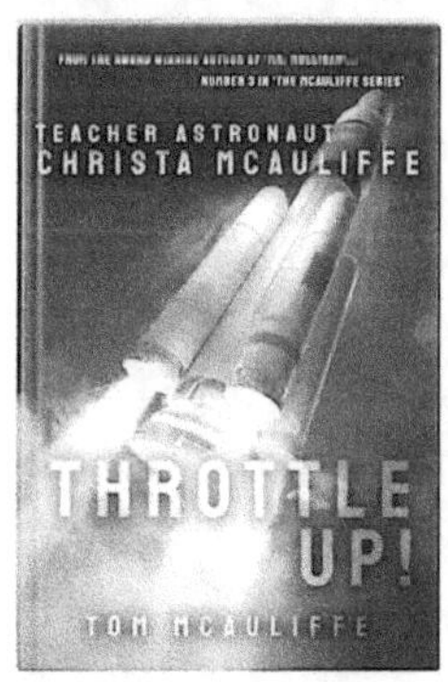
FROM THE AWARD WINNING AUTHOR OF 'MR. MULLIGAN'...
NUMBER 3 IN 'THE MCAULIFFE SERIES'
TEACHER ASTRONAUT
CHRISTA MCAULIFFE
THROTTLE
UP!
TOM MCAULIFFE

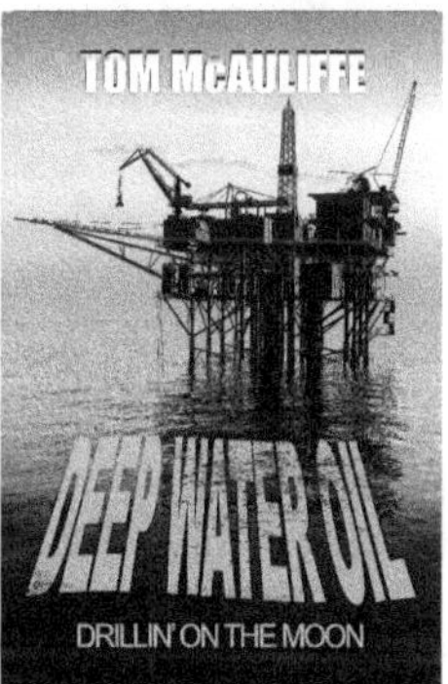
TOM McAULIFFE
DEEP WATER OIL
DRILLIN' ON THE MOON

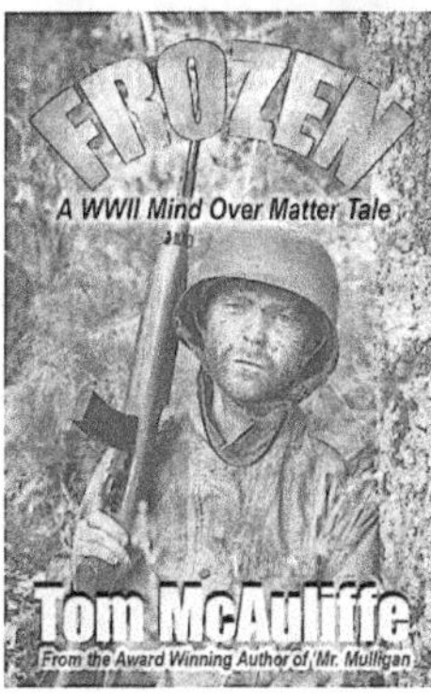
FROZEN
A WWII Mind Over Matter Tale
Tom McAuliffe
From the Award Winning Author of 'Mr. Mulligan'

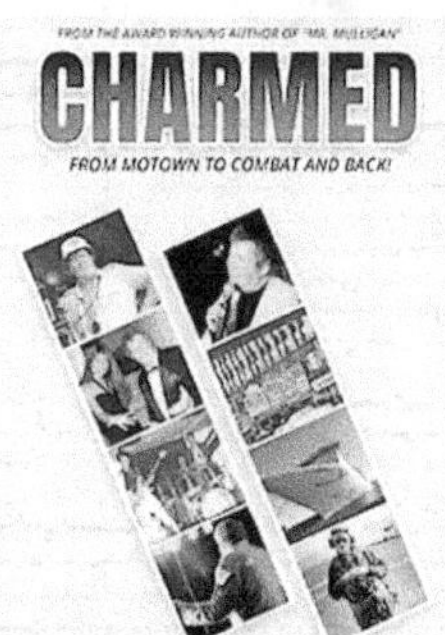
FROM THE AWARD WINNING AUTHOR OF 'MR. MULLIGAN'
CHARMED
FROM MOTOWN TO COMBAT AND BACK!
TOM MCAULIFFE

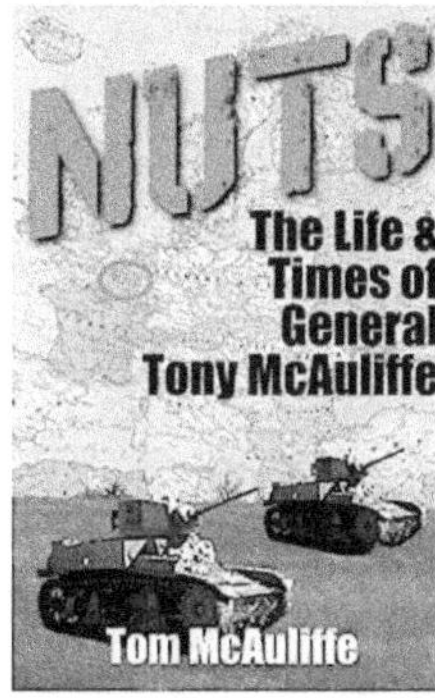
NUTS!
The Life &
Times of
General
Tony McAuliffe
Tom McAuliffe

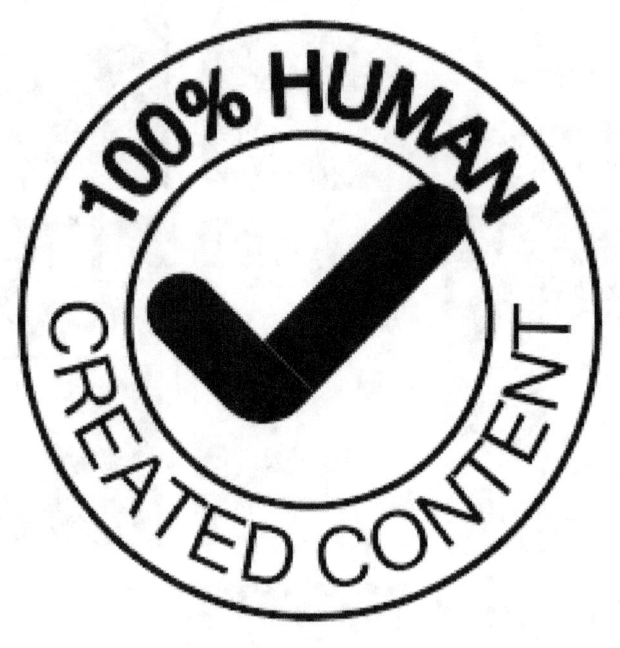

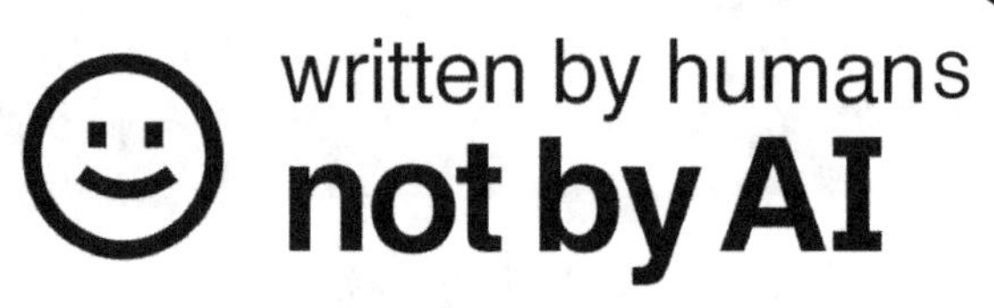
written by humans
not by AI

www.ingramcontent.com/pod-product-compliance
Lightning Source LLC
Chambersburg PA
CBHW061541120726
48001CB00004B/1656